Obsessive-Compulsive Disorder and Uncertainty

Psychodynamic Psychotherapy and Assessment in the Twenty-First Century

Series Editors: Steven Tuber, City University of New York at City College

Mission Statement

Psychodynamic Psychotherapy and Assessment establishes a milieu for the presentation of scholarly clinical work through a developmental lens. The emphasis throughout the series is on the integration of scholarship and practice through writings that are informed by both sources of learning. This domain includes works that document both evidence- based and traditional approaches within the field and applies these approaches to work with infants, children, adolescents, and adults. Efforts that link assessment to treatment are especially welcome, as are integrations between neuropsychological (brain-based) and psychological (mind or self-based) formulations about personality development and its aberrations. The impact of trauma, both chronic and acute, on the psychological lives of its victims is also an important area of study within this domain. New voices within the field are encouraged to write about the interface between the content and process of their emergent thinking and practice. In addition to the areas mentioned above, more experienced clinical scholars are encouraged to write about the supervisory process and its impact on both theory and practice. Works that focus on specific developmental processes and paradigms at points throughout the lifespan are another welcome area for contributions.

Titles in the Series

Obsessive-Compulsive Disorder and Uncertainty: Struggling with a Shadow of a Doubt, by Moshe Marcus and Steven Tuber

Psychodynamics Commencing in Early Childhood: The Case for an Additional Tripartite Complex, by Joseph Newirth

From Sign to Symbol: Transformational Processes in Psychoanalysis, Psychotherapy, and Psychology, by Marvin P. Osman

Guided Enactments in Psychoanalytic Psychotherapy: A New Look at Therapy with Adults and Children, by Sebastiano Santostefano

Obsessive-Compulsive Disorder and Uncertainty

Struggling with a Shadow of a Doubt

Moshe Marcus and Steven Tuber

LEXINGTON BOOKS
Lanham • Boulder • New York • London

Published by Lexington Books
An imprint of The Rowman & Littlefield Publishing Group, Inc.
4501 Forbes Boulevard, Suite 200, Lanham, Maryland 20706
www.rowman.com

6 Tinworth Street, London SE11 5AL, United Kingdom

British Library Cataloguing in Publication Information Available

Library of Congress Cataloging-in-Publication Data

Names: Marcus, Moshe, 1986- author. | Tuber, Steven, 1954- author.
Title: Obsessive-compulsive disorder and uncertainty : struggling with a shadow of a doubt / Moshe Marcus and Steven Tuber.
Description: Lanham : Lexington Books, [2021] | Series: Psychodynamic psychotherapy and assessment in the twenty-first century | Includes bibliographical references and index. | Summary: "Obsessive-Compulsive Disorder and Uncertainty examines the intrapsychic features of the self as it presents within OCD compulsive doubting. Moshe Marcus and Steven Tuber suggest a phenomenological framework through which to consider the interplay between the cognitive as well as affective components required to make judgments"— Provided by publisher.
Identifiers: LCCN 2021014939 (print) | LCCN 2021014940 (ebook) | ISBN 9781793646361 (cloth) | ISBN 9781793646378 (ebook) ISBN 9781793646385 (pbk)
Subjects: LCSH: Obsessive-compulsive disorder. | Compulsive behavior.
Classification: LCC RC533 .M36 2021 (print) | LCC RC533 (ebook) | DDC 616.85/227—dc23
LC record available at https://lccn.loc.gov/2021014939
LC ebook record available at https://lccn.loc.gov/2021014940

For My Family
With deep appreciation and gratitude to my wife, whose inspiring
devotion and dedication to our family made this work possible.
And to my parents, whose support and love I never had to doubt.
—Moshe Marcus

I happily dedicate my work on this book to my dear
granddaughter Charlotte, born while this book was also being
born, whose presence in my life is truly a wonder.
—Steven Tuber

Contents

Acknowledgments

It is a genuine honor for me to have had the chance to work together and share authorship with a mentor whose scholarship, teaching, and clinical training have guided countless students through their doctoral training at City College, and who embodies a synthesis of scholarship and practice that has been inspirational for me.

I would also like to acknowledge and thank the faculty of the clinical psychology program at City College for providing an environment which fosters intellectual growth and professional development.

—Moshe Marcus

I'd like to thank our Editor, Kasey Beduhn, for all her erudite and supportive work on our behalf. I especially want to acknowledge that this work is very much the thinking of the first author and I am more than delighted and honored to be a secondary part of his very original process.

—Steven Tuber

Introduction

This book aims to highlight and explicate the particular structural and intra-psychic features of the self as it presents within OCD compulsive doubting, and more broadly within OCD compulsion. Specifically, it is situated within the theoretical framework of psychodynamic theory and object-relations theory, and aims to elucidate central object-relational paradigms within OCD doubting. In order to do so, the work begins with a phenomenological overview of the nature and role of doubting within OCD, and then proceeds to suggest a broader philosophical and phenomenological framework through which to consider the interplay between both the cognitive as well as affective components required to make judgments. The development of this framework, drawn from Beiner's (1983) rendering of Kantian models of judgment, allows for a formulation of compulsive doubting linked to a sense of dis-unity and fracture within the self. This in turn allows for a consideration of the structural components of the self, and specifically, an exploration of how the self comes to integrate the demands and functions of external objects into a coherent and contiguous subjective experience. The study makes use of Schafer's (1968/1990) expositions of the processes of internalization, including identification and introjection, which suggest different permutations of self-alien and self-contiguous phenomena within the self, and which are then linked to various phenomena within OCD doubting and OCD more generally. Following Schafer, the study then considers the developmental, phenomenological, and structural frameworks of Mead, Vygotsky, and Winnicott, and further links OCD phenomena to these frameworks. Last, the book concludes with a consideration of implications for treatment.

More specifically, we will examine the qualitative, affective, and structural elements of the nature of doubt and uncertainty within Obsessive-Compulsive

Disorder (OCD), and offer some direction for a consideration of its developmental origins. We begin by attempting to delineate the role of doubt within the broader symptomatology of OCD as conceived of by the various theoretical models proposed in the literature, both empirical and qualitative.

Though the symptom presentation in OCD is fairly heterogeneous (Abramowitz et al., 2009), the disorder is broadly marked by the presence of obsessions and compulsions. According to current criteria in the *Diagnostic and Statistical Manual of Mental Disorders* (DSM-5; American Psychiatric Association, 2013), it is not necessary to have both obsessions and compulsions, as the presence of one or the other is sufficient to establish the diagnosis. Obsessions refer to persistent, intrusive, and unwanted thoughts or images that are disturbing. Compulsions are defined as repetitive behaviors (or mental acts) that are performed with a ritual quality in response to the obsessive thoughts (American Psychiatric Association, 2013). They serve to lessen the anxiety produced by the intrusion of the disturbing thoughts, and are often performed to neutralize the thoughts themselves or to forestall the occurrence of an anticipated catastrophic event. The quality of their relationship to obsessions is ritualistic, in that there is no realistic relationship between the performance of the compulsion and the reduction of the anxiety or the prevention of disaster.

According to the data presented in the DSM-5, the current 12-month prevalence of OCD is 1.2 percent within the United States, and the mean age at onset is 19.5 years. Boys typically have an earlier onset than girls, as nearly 25 percent of males diagnosed with OCD experience the onset of symptoms before they turn ten. However, the adult prevalence is higher among females. Among those patients diagnosed in childhood, 40 percent may experience remission by adulthood if untreated. The rates are different for those diagnosed as adults, where remission rates are 20 percent. As characterized by Abramowitz et al. (2009), "if untreated, the course is mainly chronic, with symptoms changing over time, often in response to life stressors." Frequently, OCD patients have comorbid conditions as well. According to the DSM-5, 76 percent of OCD patients have been diagnosed with an additional anxiety disorder, while 63 percent have been diagnosed with an additional mood disorder.

The two most common compulsions are checking and cleaning compulsions (Rachman, 2002). Checking compulsions often center around strong urges to repeatedly check for having locked the door to one's house, turned off the stove in one's kitchen, or similar tasks. Typically, the checking is done to forestall some impending harm or disaster that might befall either the patient or someone else (safety obsessions). In addition to the fear of disaster itself, these compulsions can have a moral element as well (the compulsion to retrace one's morning commute and make sure that they did not cause an accident while driving earlier in the day, as but one example), where the person is consumed by thoughts of possible guilt for having caused harm, and can only be resolved by verifying that no harm had actually occurred. Importantly, the checking does not need to be explicitly behavioral. For example, in obsessions clustered around unacceptable thoughts, a person may check in on themselves constantly by repeatedly monitoring their thoughts to determine whether or not they harbor aggressive wishes towards a loved one.

Cleaning compulsions often revolve around contamination obsessions, in which a person experiences an intense and exaggerated fear of contamination, either of something "real," such as pathogens and disease, or something idiosyncratic. Compulsions that arise in relationship to these fears, such as frequent and repetitive hand washing, are intended to address either actual (perceived) contamination, or the possibility of having been contaminated. Taken together, compulsions then "are associated with doubting and indecisiveness" (Rachman, 2002, p. 627), though this association is stronger for checking compulsions than for cleaning compulsions (Rachman, 2002). This association is manifest in two forms. Most directly, in checking compulsions, the checking is a direct attempt to resolve the doubt; repeatedly checking the position of a lock is intended to verify that it is indeed in the correct position. Importantly, though, compulsive checking does not usually result in the termination of doubting and uncertainty, even when the checking is repeated many times. This is an important and interesting element of the symptomatology, and one that the various models and theories of compulsive checking have attempted to address. These will be described in more detail in the course of this chapter.

The second manifestation of this association is less direct, and concerns the nature of the obsessive thoughts themselves. That is, the anticipation of any given harm or disaster is itself reflective of an uncertainty or confusion surrounding the likelihood, or probability, of the event occurring. It is seemingly the mere possibility of disaster and harm which generates the anxiety (I might have left the stove on), and the concomitant compulsion (Aardema & O'Connor, 2012).

We turn now to an overview of the contemporary empirical literature surrounding compulsive checking, maintaining a focus on the role and nature of the doubting and uncertainty that are operative in checking compulsions. Early behavioral models have focused on the connection between compulsions and obsessions, and have explicated the behavioral factors reinforcing compulsions; because compulsions dispel (at least temporarily) the anxiety engendered by intrusive obsessional thoughts, they become reinforced as the patient begins to rely on them as a primary mechanism for dealing with obsessive anxiety. However, cognitive and neuropsychological models have more explicitly intended to take up the nature and causes of the doubt at the center of obsessive thoughts, and which fuels compulsive behavior. Much of this research and theory has focused on compulsive checking, and we will begin by outlining the various models and mechanisms proposed to account for the significant features of the symptomatology.

Hezel and McNally (2016), in their review of cognitive biases and deficits in OCD, trace the broad development of cognitive and metacognitive models of the disorder. They begin their account with the CBT model proposed by Salkovskis (1985), who argued that intrusive thoughts should be understood not as negative automatic thoughts, but as cognitive stimuli, and maintained that it is the interpretations and attributions made in response to these thoughts that explains both the nature and origin of the symptomatology. Salkovskis argues that intrusive thoughts are not in and of themselves a feature of OCD; rather, most people are likely to experience intrusive and disturbing thoughts from time to time. What distinguishes OCD, and explains the obsessional quality of the thoughts, is not the thoughts themselves but cognitive features surrounding them.

Specifically, Salkovskis (1985) suggests a model in which intrusive thoughts can trigger two possible reactions. The first possible kind of reaction is dismissal, such that the person believes that the thoughts have no particular significance or salience, and simply moves on. Salkovskis theorizes that this is the way most people (in the non-clinical population) deal with their intrusive thoughts. However, the second kind of possible reaction derives from attributions of salience and significance: "if ... they believe that thoughts of this kind might have important implications, then automatic thoughts would be expected to arise as a function of the strength of the beliefs concerned" (Salkovskis, 1985, p. 578). These kinds of automatic thoughts often revolve around the notion of an "inflated responsibility" (as characterized by Hezel & McNally, 2016), in which the person experiences themselves as bearing some responsibility for these thoughts. The responsibility can take different forms, among these are: conflations of thought and action, in which a thought about an action is equivalent to performing it; that passivity in reaction to these thoughts is equivalent to wishing for them to happen; and that one is responsible for controlling his thoughts and preventing unwanted thoughts. The perceived responsibility for these thoughts leads to a compulsion to "neutralize" (Salkovskis, 1985, p. 578) the potential harm or blame through rituals or "undoing" actions, which does lessen the anxiety. This thereby reinforces the efficacy of the compulsions, and also prevents the opportunity to learn that the thoughts are in fact meaningless.

In addition to the distortions suggested by Salkovskis et al., Hezel and McNally (2016) also note three additional dispositions that have been suggested as critical to the formation of OCD symptoms. These are the overestimation of threat bias, the construct of intolerance of ambiguity, and the focus on perfectionism. Overestimation of threat refers to the tendency to which someone might appraise the possibility of impending harm, introduced by an intrusive thought, as being significantly much higher or more realistic than it actually is. This, in addition to the sense of "inflated responsibility" to prevent harm, works to keep the individual experiencing intrusive thoughts in a state of hyper-vigilance against a fairly continuous barrage of perceived imminent threats, which are in turn to be neutralized by compulsions.

Intolerance for ambiguity refers to the intense levels of distress experienced by individuals during situations of uncertainty and doubt. As described by Buhr and Dugas (2009), individuals with low tolerance for ambiguity find the experience of uncertainty and doubt highly aversive, and are often compelled to "engage in futile attempts to control or eliminate uncertainty" (Buhr & Dugas, 2009, as cited by Hezel & McNally, 2016, p. 223). It is theorized then that the intensity of compulsive urges, especially for checking behaviors, is contributed to by the heightened sensitivity and low tolerance that patients with OCD are thought to maintain with regard to uncertainties generated by obsessive thoughts (Tolin et al., 2003). Interestingly though, Tolin et al. (2003) suggest further that CBT treatment for OCD should incorporate this finding into clinical practice, and aim to reduce patients' intolerance of ambiguity (IU) as a core element of the treatment. While the rationale seems clear, and their research has seemingly established a link between IU and OCD, there is something curious about this suggestion, in that it seemingly prioritizes the tolerance of uncertainty over the development of certainty itself. As we will see, many have conceptualized an inability to experience certainty as one of the core symptoms of OCD. Surely, in the instance of compulsive checking, such as repeatedly making sure that a door is locked, the issue seems not to be the tolerance of uncertainty, but the attainment of certainty where it is warranted. We will return to explore this point more fully when we turn to a fuller consideration of the role of doubting in OCD.

Perfectionism refers to the belief that one must always meet exceptionally high standards (across domains; whether morally, academically, professionally, etc.), and that failure to meet these high standards, in any instance, indicates a more global and characterological failure. As described by Hezel and McNally (2016), the link between perfectionism and OCD takes place among three main pathways. The first is that it is thought to play a role in raising the degree to which one might expect to maintain control over their thoughts and their environments. Additionally, perfectionistic tendencies are thought to increase the sense of responsibility that individuals may feel for negative events and negative thoughts. And last, perfectionism is related to the phenomenological construct at the heart of much of OCD symptomatology, termed Not Just Right Experiences (NJREs). OCD patients often report "an inner drive that is connected with a wish to have things perfect, absolutely certain, or completely under control" (Rasmussen & Eisen, 1992, cited by

Coles et al., 2003, p. 682). Until this state is experienced, patients have a sense that things are not "just right," and are thought to repetitively continue their compulsions until they experience a feeling of "just right." Importantly, Coles et al. (2003) note that NJRE's represent an additional and distinct catalyst for compulsive behavior (aside from the forestalling of catastrophe).

As Hezel and McNally conclude, studies (Taylor et al., 2010, as cited by Hezel & McNally, 2016) have shown a relationship among these patterns of dysfunctional thoughts and the symptoms of OCD, suggesting the validity of the cognitive models described above. However, further theorizing about the nature of OCD thinking has led to the development of the metacognitive model, which postulates that there is a substantive distinction between beliefs about the world and the self (such as overestimation of harm and perfectionism biases), and beliefs about the nature of one's thoughts themselves. According to the metacognitive model, it is this second category of beliefs that is the catalytic mechanism for the development of OCD.

As described by Hansmeir et al. (2016), the model suggests two levels of metacognitive beliefs. At the first level are fusion beliefs. Thought-Action Fusion is the belief that thinking about a given action will by necessity lead one to carry out the action, even in the absence of any desire to do so. Thought-Event Fusion is the belief that the presence of a thought concerning an event (thinking about having run someone over with a car, for example) demonstrates that the event in fact happened, and the thought is in fact a memory. Thought-Object Fusion is the belief that thinking about an object can have an effect on the object itself (thinking that an object has been contaminated will actually effect a transfer of the contamination to the object). An intrusive thought serves as a trigger for these first-level beliefs, which in turn trigger a second level of beliefs concerning rituals. These beliefs include assumptions about the necessity and effectiveness of relevant rituals (which then trigger the performance of the compulsions) and "subjective stop signals" which provide an idiosyncratic monitoring mechanism providing the feedback alerting the patient when it is alright to conclude the performance of the ritual (when the function of the ritual has been fully attained). While the metacognitive model acknowledges the validity of existing CBT models and the critical role of dysfunctional beliefs, it emphasizes the role of metacognitive beliefs that are superordinate to these dysfunctional beliefs. Studies (cited by Hezel & McNally, 2016; Hansmeier et al., 2016) have shown that these metacognitive beliefs do predict OCD symptoms, and do so even when controlling for OCD dysfunctional beliefs.

While these models (the cognitive and metacognitive) have focused more broadly on the role of appraisals in response to intrusive thoughts and the pathway from obsession to compulsion, other approaches have attempted to elucidate the peculiar nature of the mentation within the context of compulsive checking. More specifically, these approaches have attempted to explain how it can be that OCD patients experience uncertainty and doubt surrounding seemingly mundane and simple tasks (such as having locked the door), whereas most people have no difficulty feeling and being quite certain about these (and the certainty seems warranted). There have been two main approaches to these issues. The first of these has focused on identifying potential neuropsychological deficits within OCD patients that might provide a compelling account for these perplexing experiences. The second approach maintains that there are no identifiable global deficits in neuropsychological functioning, but rather, the individual patient's habits of mind can themselves produce effects on memory and attention that lead to the experiences of doubt and uncertainty, thereby simulating neuropsychological deficits, but not deriving from an organic source.

The relevant neuropsychological deficits are thought to present in two primary domains, memory and executive functioning. Given the particular nature of compulsive checking, researchers have naturally wondered about the possibility of memory impairments within OCD patients and whether these might provide an explanation for the particular features of OCD symptomatology. Potential deficits in the domain of response inhibition are thought to play a role both regarding the inhibition of compulsive behavior (in the sense that patients feel a need to perform an action that they would like to inhibit), as well as the inability to inhibit obsessive thoughts (Chamberlain et al., 2005). Additional attentional processes are also thought to play a role in OCD symptoms (Muller & Roberts, 2005), as a heightened sensitivity to emotionally salient stimuli (especially those coded as threatening) would lead to increased and preferential attention awarded to thoughts of harm and doubt. Concerning the overall effects of potential executive functioning deficits, a recent meta-analysis performed by Abramovitch et al. (2013) noted considerable inconsistency between studies, but did find small to moderate effect sizes across a broad range of executive functioning domains[1].

That being said, however, a few issues have been raised concerning the body of neuropsychological deficits. The first issue concerns the clinical significance of these findings. As Abramovitch et al. (2013) argue, an analysis of the effect sizes in their meta-analysis indicates that while discrepancies between OCD patients and controls are significant statistically across domains, the degree of impairment present in OCD patients falls below conventional cutoffs for impairment used in clinical neuropsychology. As such, they conclude that it is difficult to argue that these deficits should be seen as primary catalysts for the development and etiology of OCD symptoms.

Secondly, some of these deficits may be explained by other factors, including metacognitive processes. Notably, two additional metacognitive elements are seen as having particular importance to the issue of potential memory impairments in compulsive checking. The first of these is the phenomenon described as cognitive self-consciousness (CSC) (Janeck et al., 2003, as cited by Hezel & McNally, 2016), which is a tendency to monitor one's own thoughts. Studies (Exner et al., 2009) have shown that the increased cognitive load generated by this self-monitoring can cause impairments in memory, which, given the presence of CSC in OCD patients, might thereby account for the appearance of memory deficits in OCD subjects (Exner et al., 2009, as cited by Hezel et al., 2016). The second metacognitive element is that of memory confidence. Patients with OCD are theorized to have lower confidence in their memories, which might account for checking behaviors even in the absence of a genuine deficit or memory impairment. Critically though, it has also been found that repeated checking causes both a decrease in memory confidence (Tolin et al., 2001), as well as shifts in the nature of memory, decreasing the acuity of specific details within recall of an episodic memory and prompting reliance on more generalized heuristic recall strategies (van den Hout & Kundt, 2003).

Additionally, in a more recent review of neuropsychological functioning within OCD, Abramovitch and Cooperman (2015) argue for a state-based model of neuropsychological deficits, in which the "overflow of obsessive thoughts overloads the executive system in a way which is similar to having numerous open programs on a personal computer that overloads the RAM memory . . . . This overload may then result in neuropsychological deficits in OCD" (p. 31). As such, it is the nature of the disorder itself that generates these deficits, which are not pre-existing and therefore do not have much explanatory power. Accordingly, Abramovitch et al. argue that these deficits should recede as the symptoms attenuate, and cite studies (including Voderholzer et al., 2013) showing improvement in neuropsychological performance following treatment, though they acknowledge that the evidence is inconclusive.

However, a broader, more fundamental critique can be made of these approaches. As Dar et al. (2000) argue, the phenomenology of OCD doubting goes beyond the issue of memory:

> This apparent lack of confidence in OC checkers may not necessarily be restricted to memory judgment. In fact, a striking phenomenon in these patients is their inability to feel certain even in the face of seemingly clear and unambiguous evidence. For example, an OC checker may turn the key in the lock over and over again without being able to convince himself or herself that the door has in fact been locked, even though he or she can plainly see that the key is in the proper position, hear it engaging, and feel the lock snapping. (p. 673)

For Dar et al. it is the *inability to feel certain* that is at the center of OCD symptomatology. This view has also been expressed in earlier research and thinking about OCD. Freud (1909) famously discusses the disorder in his presentation of the Rat Man case. In brief, obsessional-neuroses have their origin in love-hate ambivalences that develop early in childhood. The hatred and aggression are repressed in the unconscious, where they persist as aggressive and sadistic desires, while the fundamental ambivalence of love and hate remains unresolved. Thus, the patient is left with "an intense love opposed by an almost equally powerful hatred, and is at the same time inseparably bound up with it" (Freud, 1909, p. 241). As such "the immediate consequence is certain to be a partial paralysis of the will and an incapacity for coming to a decision upon any of those actions for which love ought to provide the motive power" (Freud, 1909, p. 241).

For Freud, the disorder is then marked by two features, doubt and compulsion:

> Doubt corresponds to the patient's internal perception of his own indecision, which, in consequence of the inhibition of his love by his hatred, takes possession of him in the face of every intended action. The doubt is in reality a doubt of his own love. (p. 241)

Because the patient's own aggressive and sadistic impulses towards the love-object are defended against, the feeling of ambivalence is displaced onto virtually everything else, creating a "paralysis of will" (Freud, 1909, p. 241). The compulsions arise out of the patient's need to resolve his incapacitating doubts, and derive their particular potency and insistent quality from the "dammed up energy" (Freud, 1909, p. 244) that has been unable to discharge itself during the course of the indecision.

Reed (1976, as cited by Frost & Shows, 1993), working within a cognitive and information-processing framework, also takes the position that doubt and indecisiveness are at the core of OCD symptomatology. Reed asserts that indecisiveness and doubt "have been stressed as central characteristics of obsessive-compulsive disorder by practically every psychiatric authority who has written on the topic" (Reed, 1976, as quoted by Frost & Shows, 1993, p. 683). In Reed's (1977) conceptualization, the central element involved in compulsive checking is the diminished or impaired ability to reach conclusions. Specifically, according to Reed, this derives from a "functional impairment in the spontaneous organization and integration of experience" (Reed, 1968, p. 382, as cited by Szechtman & Woody, 2004, p. 112). This impairment in turn causes the OCD patient to "impose exaggerated structure on his experience" (Reed, 1976, p. 443). This excessively formal "artificial overstructuring" (Reed, 1976, p. 443) of experiences, leaves patients without an organically constructed schematic for navigating and making sense of their own experiences. As such, they are left without the essential referents for making decisions, and are left with a persistent sense of uncertainty and doubt[2].

Nonetheless, there is a crucial distinction between the conceptualization suggested by Reed, and that suggested by Dar et al. (2000). Szechtman and Woody (2004) criticize Reed's model for being too cognitive; while they concur with the essential categorization of OCD doubting as a failure to attain closure, they argue that "If it were indeed true that patients suffered from a broken cognitive module (used for classification of information), then they should have profound intellectual difficulty with very many everyday tasks. Such is not the case, however" (Szechtman & Woody, 2014, p. 113). Rather, they propose a model that involves an affective process, not a cognitive one, that is defined by a neurobiological mechanism triggered by the presence of "subjective conviction" (p. 115), and "a feeling of knowing" (p. 111). Subjective affective certainty signals goals attainment and therefore inhibits motivation for task completion. Szechtman and Woody propose that OCD patients are not capable of generating this "endogenous" signal (p. 116), and as such find themselves in states of perpetual doubt and with a persistent sense that something is not right. Importantly, Szechtman and Woody locate this model within a proposed "security motivation system" (p. 111), acti-vated by the potential harm and perceived threat associated with obsessive thoughts. This proposed model, and the distinction between objective and affective certainty, is consistent with the criticism leveled by Dar et al. (2000) on contemporary cognitive models of OCD.

Similarly, the same criticism (and distinction) can be made regarding Inference Based Therapy (IBT), a variant of cognitive treatment for OCD. As described by Aardema and O'Connor (2012), the treatment is based on the IBA (Inference Based Approach) model, which maintains that OCD obsessions result from a fundamental cognitive error (an "inferential confu-sion," Aardema et al., 2012, p. 855) in which too much credence is given to hypothetical possibilities (obsessive thoughts which manifest as "maybe" thoughts), which causes an erosion of confidence in one's own senses. The therapy therefore aims to correct this excessive and unwarranted inference of meaningful material from mere entertainment of unlikely hypotheticals. However, this model assumes that the doubt, while central to symptomatol-ogy, is purely cognitive and informational in nature, and seemingly does not properly account for instances in which there is no missing information, such as the lock turning example raised by the critique in Dar et al. (2000).

In order to test their theory that OCD checkers fail to experience affective certainty even in the context of "clear and unambiguous evidence" (Dar et al., 2000, p. 673), Dar et al. (2000) administered a general knowledge question-naire to OCD compulsive checkers and asked them to rate their confidence level after each response. The questionnaire was comprised of 100 items testing general knowledge, and had two choices for each question. The questions themselves were derived from psychometric examinations provided by the National Institute for Testing and Evaluation in Israel. After each item, the questionnaire asked participants to rate how confident they were that their choice was correct, using a scale of 5–100 percent, with 5 percent increments. Dar et al. found that relative to actual performance, compulsive checkers were significantly less confident in their knowledge than healthy controls.

Accordingly, Dar et al. (2000) concluded that affective certainty is independent of informational knowledge, and that OC checkers are differentiated by a diminished ability to feel confident about what it is that they actually do know (in an informational sense). They raise two related questions about the nature of their finding: the first is whether this diminished confidence is a cause or an effect of OCD symptomatology, and the second question is how to account for the phenomenon; namely, what mechanisms are responsible for causing this global lack of confidence? Interestingly, with regard to the second question, they propose the presence of a "disconfirmation bias," "which generates a search for evidence that might undermine OC checkers' confidence in their hypotheses" (Dar et al., 2000, p. 677). It seems important to point out, that proposed mechanism seems to be fundamentally cognitive in nature. This seemingly then is tangential to the essential point of the study, which was to address how it can be that OCD patients experience a lack of certainty even where the informational context leaves no room for ambiguity and uncertainty.

Lazarov et al. (2010), building on Dar's previous work as well as "feeling of knowing" models including the model developed by Szechtman et al. (2004), proposed that in the absence of "feelings of knowing," patients with OCD rely on "external proxies" as a "substitute for the internal state that the individual perceives as more easily discernible or less ambiguous, such as rules, procedures, behaviors or environmental stimuli" (Lazarov et al., 2012, p. 557). This model is referred to as the "seeking-proxies-for-internal-states" (SPIS) hypothesis. Importantly, as Lazarov et al. (2012) note, in contrast to Szechtman's model which focused on the context of threat and harm-initiated processes, SPIS maintains that patients with OCD have a more global diminishment in their ability to access and infer internal states; these states are not restricted to those activated by heightened responsibility or threat salience. Rather, OCD patients can experience a "lack of subjective conviction" (Lazarov et al., 2012, p. 557) which may be present "in any area of human functioning where doubt and uncertainty emerge" (Lazarov et al., 2012, p. 557). These areas include affective states (including attraction, to which we will return shortly) and cognitive functioning, including uncertainty within the context of memory (which thereby accommodates and incorporates the findings about metacognitive elements in reduced memory confidence). That is to say, patients with OCD are prone to experience uncertainty and doubt about their own internal states, and have difficulty definitively identifying them. As a coping strategy, these patients develop and rely on rule-based schematics (termed "proxies") to settle their own uncertainty.[3] Interestingly, the SPIS model proposes that compulsive behaviors, rather than the byproduct of a certainty-seeking process that fails to terminate conclusively, are themselves a "proxy" for internal states, such that the formal action of washing one's hands is a proxy for an internal feeling state of "cleanliness" which is not readily attainable.

Among the studies performed by Lazarov et al. (2010), was a study done within a biofeedback paradigm relating to muscle tension, though the feedback was actually false. They found that OCD subjects were misled by the false feedback at a significantly higher rate than control subjects, from which they inferred that the OCD subjects were relying more heavily on the external cues provided through the feedback than on their own internal feel for their degree of muscle tension. Lazarov et al. (2010) do raise the question as to what mechanisms contribute to this diminished access to internal states, but again seem to propose the presence of metacognitive elements.

It seems important to point out that the diminished access to internal states proposed by Lazarov et al. is seemingly different than the more amorphous and diffuse confusion and chaos experienced within the context of personality disorders, and especially BPD, where an inability to regulate affect is thought to be connected to poor insight and reflective functioning about internal affect states (see, for instance, Yeomans et al., 2015). Rather, what seems to be happening here are two different but related processes. The first is a difficulty with reconciling ambivalent (as described by Freud, 1909) and conflicting (though stable and well-defined) feelings about a given situation into an integrated total, unified, and coherent experience, in which either one of the poles of the ambivalence becomes dominant, or a third possibility presents itself that resolves the ambivalence. The second process is that doubt functions like one of the poles of the ambivalent situation, such that there is ambivalence and uncertainty about whether certainty has been sufficiently achieved. It is still a relatively binary choice between affirming the existence of an internal state, based on any given set of internal cues, or rejecting the existence of a given internal state, based on the absence (or presence) of a (sometimes different) set of cues.

This becomes clearer when considering Doron et al.'s (2014) consideration of Relationship OCD (ROCD).[4] They present the following clinical vignette as an illustration of the phenomenon:

> David, a 32-year-old business consultant living with his partner for three months, enters my office and describes his problem: "I've been in a relationship for a year, but I can't stop thinking about whether this is the right relationship

for me. I see other woman [sic] on the street or on Facebook and I can't stop thinking whether I will be happier with them, or feel more in love with them. I ask my friends what they think. I check what I feel for her over and over again, whether I remember her face, whether I think about her enough. I know I love my partner, but I have to check and recheck. I feel depressed. I can't go on like this." (p. 169)

Thus, the condition is marked by obsessive and intrusive aversive thoughts, in which a person is compelled to repeatedly engage in mental checking in an attempt to resolve a persistent state of doubt and uncertainty regarding their own internal affective state. This doubt is not diffuse; it is not as if David is experiencing strong emotions that he cannot explain, while feeling disoriented and confused. Rather, he experiences himself as stuck in a binary; between affirming his affection for his partner based on the given set of factors which created and maintain the reaction, or between determining that his feelings of affection are not sufficiently strong, based either on latent (relatively unacknowledged) misgivings and ambivalences, or on his interest in other women.

Last, it bears mention that recent research on the construct of indecisiveness has shown an effect of indecisiveness on quality of life in patients diagnosed with OCD (Taillefer et al., 2016). Defined as "the general tendency to experience decision difficulties" (Rassin, 2007, as cited by Taillefer et al., 2016, p. 92), it has been suggested that indecisiveness has trait-like attributes (see Germeijs & Verschueren, 2011, for their overview and findings) with effects that are independent and distinct from Big 5 personality traits (though appropriately related to such traits as neuroticism), and thus quite naturally seems to be relevant to OCD symptomatology. As such, this finding serves as well to point to the centrality of doubt and uncertainty within OCD symptomatology.

Summing up our overview of the literature, there are two central points that need to be made. The first is that one of the central elements of OCD is the lack of *affective certainty* about external and internal worlds. What remains unaddressed is both the developmental trajectory for this kind of certainty, as well as a fuller developmental consideration for what has likely gone awry in those diagnosed with OCD. The second point here is that what is being described is an affective process, as the experience of certainty is generated by mechanisms and processes that while connected to cognition, are also to a significant degree outside the domain of cognition. As Dar et al. (2000) describe, in the case of the obsessive repeatedly turning the lock to check that it has been done properly, there is no role for cognition because no new information can be gleaned from environmental stimuli. Rather, the experience of affective certainty is dependent on what is being done with the information already present in the mind. Given that this is the case, what we are really doing is talking about the process of judgment, in the sense that a *determination* is made about information that is already given. We therefore need to consider a fuller model of judgment to make sense of the process as it usually happens, and what is going awry in OCD symptomatology. We turn to Kant's model of reflective judgment because of its integration of affect into the model of judgment, and its emphasis on the unity of judgment. Additionally, Kantian models of judgment, as we will suggest, offer a bridge to psychodynamic correlates revolving around object-relations, superego development, and the process of internalization. We turn next to begin our outline of Kantian models of judgment.

NOTES

1. See Leopold and Backenstrass (2015) for an argument that EF deficits in checkers are much more pronounced than in washers, and their effects in the former group are therefore likely underestimated because of studies that have included both checkers and washers.

2. Reed goes on to add additional steps and levels to his model, incorporating additional cognitive and metacognitive elements. See Frost and Shows (1993) for a brief summation.

3. Though Lazarov et al. primarily describe "proxies" as ruled-based schematics, they also do seem to suggest that the term also includes reassurance-seeking behaviors, such that one may seek to elicit and rely on the assurances and determinations made by others because of the absence of an internal state of "knowing." See Lazarov et al. (2012): "SPIS conceptualization can be used to explain to patients how these doubts and uncertainties can lead to compensatory compulsive behaviors such as excessive reliance on norms, rules and rituals and *to seeking external validation from others*" (p. 562) (italics added).

4. For a full overview of the model, including its links to cognitive models as well as attachment theory, see Doron et al. (2014).

Chapter 1

A Kantian Model of Judgment

Kant's theory of judgment is important to us for two reasons. The first is that he takes up the question of judgment not only through a philosophical consideration of language and content (though his approach to content is important to us as well, as we will see) but because he posits and elucidates the various mental processes and components through which judgment happens and is possible. Therefore, it readily lends itself as a tool and building block through which to model a psychological account of judgment. Additionally, Kant's emphasis on judgment as a central component and critical capacity through which the self expresses its full unity and autonomy is particularly germane to those for whom difficulty with judgment is a central part of their experience, that is, those suffering with OCD. This inability to come to ordinary judgments is often experienced within the context of compulsive symptoms that create a psychological climate that is hostile to and inhibits the subjective experience of freedom. We begin then with an overview[1] of Kant's model and corresponding meta-psychology, with special attention given to highlighting the elements of his theory that are of particular relevance and benefit to our study.

We begin by noting that for Kant, cognition consists of basic faculties and complex faculties.[2] The two basic faculties identified by Kant as the building blocks for more complex forms of cognition are "understanding" (*Verstand*), and "sensibility" (*Sinnlichkeit*). The former is the faculty that refers to the element of "concepts" (which we will explain more fully below) as well as the mental processes involved in logical and discursive reasoning. The latter refers to intuitions, sense perception, and mental imagery. For Kant, "concepts" refer both to the latent ("a priori," in Kantian terminology) schemata and logical rules used by the mind to organize and systematize mental representation, as well as the range of actual representations organized and systematized according to logical rules and expressed in logical form. The systematized representations themselves can be understood as "concepts" in the sense that they represent a databank of conceptual knowledge, from which deductions and inferences can be made following the rules of formal logic. Indeed, for Kant, the a priori concepts play a role in the process of apperception in that they facilitate classification and organize the perceptions of objects.[3] Intuitions, the primary element of "sensibility," are by definition non-conceptual. They are sense-related object-representations and can be understood broadly as the mental byproduct of an object's impingement on the senses.

These two basic faculties, understanding and sensibility, are in turn mediated and regulated by two additional faculties, "imagination" (*Einbildungskraft*) and "reason" (*Vernunft*). Imagination, broadly, is the vehicle through which the mind can act on and make use of sensible material (cognitions and representations),[4] both in terms of accessing sensible impressions in the absence of concrete perception, as well as filling in crucial elements to make perception more meaningful. In terms of the former function, the imagination is responsible for reconstituting a perceptual intuition even when the object itself is no longer present. In terms of the latter, the imagination situates perceptual intuitions within time and space. The perception of time and space, according to Kant, is not derived directly from sensory experience, in that the "impingement" of an object upon the sensory system is not by itself sufficient to generate a full account of its temporal and spatial orientation. These are filled in by a super-sensory capacity; space and time are a priori forms for the organization of sense data, and Kant identifies the imagination as the faculty capable of generating the constitution and synthesis of these gestalt elements. For example, an infant's sensory system approximates in essential ways that of an adult's, yet from what we understand infants do not possess the requisite intellectual development to form what we understand as a "concept of time."[5]

Additionally, the imagination also serves to provide more specific forms of schematic rules for applying the more general concepts to any given object. For example, a child who has not yet acquired object constancy and sees a magic trick of a disappearing coin perceives the coin to be "gone," whereas an adult perceives the coin as "hidden," and wants to understand how the trick was performed. Importantly, it is also capable of generating new mental imagery, reflected in the common usage of the word "imagination," in that the mind can conjure an image of something that it has not yet seen. Essentially, it serves to fill the gap between concrete and abstract, and drives mentation forward beyond cognition of sensation, to make the jump from what is there to what is not there, and conversely, from what is not there to what is there.

Similarly, the faculty of reason allows for higher-order thinking by facilitating logical inferences (in this sense, also moving thought beyond basic cognition), and more importantly, seeking to create a coherent systematization of all existing cognitive material. Additionally, it is active in the formation and implementation of higher-order and more complex concepts necessary for moral and practical judgment and reasoning. As such, the faculty of reason also provides regulative ideas to facilitate the formation of moral and epistemological principles.

Having laid out the broad elements of Kant's model of the mind, we can now trace how he defines the parameters of judgment as well as models its mechanisms and function. For Kant, judgment happens through the faculty of apperception, whereby the mind binds together

> all the otherwise uncoordinated sub-acts and sub-contents of intuition, conceptualization, imagination, and reason, via apperception or rational self-consciousness, for the purpose of generating a single cognitive product, the judgment, under the overarching pure concepts of the understanding or categories, thereby fully integrating the several distinct cognitive faculties and their several distinct sorts of representational information, and thereby constituting a single rational human animal. (Hanna, 2017)

Thus, the power of judgment is the self's conscious affirmation of its own unified apperception, such that it generates a cognition of *"I think"* (*Ich denke*). The form of this cognition is propositional, in that judgments are "an act of logical predication whereby a concept is applied to a thing, as expressed by the copula 'is' or 'are'" (Hanna, 2017, citing Kant). As such, Kant arrives at a definition for judgment that "the power of judgment is the faculty of subsuming under rules, i.e, of determining whether something stands under a given rule or not" (Kant, cited by Hanna, 2017). The term "subsumption" is critical to Kant's account. To clarify briefly, this refers to the organization and systematization of perception into apperception, in the sense of rendering a given percept into an intelligible object by associating it with categories, schemata, and concepts.

This definition is important to us for a few reasons. The first, by emphasizing propositional content of judgment, Kant is moving away from judgments as merely evaluative feelings, since for him they center on an intentional act; judgments are not merely passive reactions to experienced stimuli. Thus, by emphasizing the "binding function" (Hanna, 2017) of judgment, Kant's account highlights the very dilemma of ambivalence, in which judgment, qua "judgment," is being hindered and blocked. As such, Kant's account allows for a direct connection between ambivalence and what might clinically be understood as a crisis of judgment. While others have argued that judgments are merely a "representation of a relation between two concepts" (Hanna, 2017, citing Kant's account of the Port Royalists, a philosophical group of logicians interested in the nature of concepts in the aftermath of Descartes), this definition would not allow us to connect judgment to ambivalence; each pole of an ambivalent attitude might simply be understood to constitute its own proto-judgment, positing an independent "representation of a relation between concepts." By insisting on the unified nature of a judgment, however, we are able to connect judgment to ambivalence, in that it is no longer viable to maintain that each pole of the ambivalent attitude constitutes its own independent judgment; "judgment," in fact, could only be understood as an ultimate determination, that is, a choice between the two poles. Importantly, emphasizing the "binding function" of judgment and its unified nature highlight the problematic nature of the crisis of judgment that happens during compulsive doubting and paralyzing ambivalence.

Having outlined broadly the basic mechanics of Kantian judgment, we turn our attention now to Kant's treatment of aesthetic judgment, and trace the broad outlines of his model.[6] As we have mentioned, for Kant, the essence of judgment is the "thinking [of] the particular under the universal" (Kant, cited by Ginsborg, 2014), as constituted in the grammatical and syntactic form "an object x is a category y." In his Critique of Judgment, Kant distinguishes between two kinds of judgments, "determining" (*bestimmend*) and "reflecting" (*reflektierend*) judgments. In determinative judgments, the pertinent concept or universal is already given, and a determination is made to subsume[7] a given particular under the relevant (and corresponding) universal. For instance, a judgment that a given object belongs to the particular category of "table." However, in reflective judgments, the appropriate universal is not given, and the mind must generate from within itself an appropriate universal or concept under which to subsume the given particular. While the particular parameters of what constitutes a "reflective judgment" will be described below, Kant's development of this type of judgment is primarily in relation to aesthetic judgments of beauty and hence our rationale for focusing on it here.

Though reflective judgments are distinct from determinative judgments, reflective judgment itself is at times operative within cognitive processes.[8] For instance, reflective judgment "is responsible for various tasks associated with empirical scientific inquiry" (Ginsborg, 2014) including taxonomy and the formation of scientific theories. In these processes, the reflective element is the generation of a universal to create a systematization of nature.

Indeed, given this last function of reflective judgments, Kant introduces the notion of teleological judgments, in which the mind posits (and perceives nature according to certain) fundamental assumptions about purpose and ends. Namely, that nature and living organisms possess function and purposiveness. While a full outline of teleological judgments falls outside the scope of our needs, it is important to note briefly that for Kant, the very existence of life, and living matter, cannot be explained purely mechanistically and must make recourse to teleological explanations about the purpose of there being life and living organisms. In fact, according to Kant, reflecting on the "ends" and purposes of natural life suggests to us the existence of an intelligent being who is the cause of nature, "and drives us to seek a theology" (Kant, as quoted by Ginsborg, 2014) to account for the nature of God and the purpose of man. For Kant, this itself is based on a moral teleology in which man is the final purpose of nature due to the fact that humans, among all creatures, can stand outside of nature and make use of it. As we will see, the fact that man stands outside of nature will be important to a later consideration of the parameters of reflective judgment.

As we have mentioned, Kant's account of reflective judgment also includes judgments that rely on the input of feelings, and particularly, the feelings of pleasure and displeasure. Kant describes three such classes of judgment: judgments of the agreeable, judgments of beauty (also referred to as judgments of taste, or "Jt"), and judgments of the sublime. The distinctions between the first two are of particular concern to our account, and will emerge from Kant's account of the defining features of aesthetic judgment, in what are known as the "four moments." We will go through them here, and will be following closely Ginsborg's (2014) summary.

The first point is that Jt are based on a "disinterested pleasure." In essence, this contains two points. Saying that something is beautiful is different than saying that a given object is green, because the latter is based solely on perception and sensation, while the former makes recourse to a subjective experience of the object. As such, Jt are differentiated from cognitive judgments. However, while the subjective experience is the feeling of pleasure, this pleasure is different than the one operative in judgments of the agreeable, since it does not depend on the subject's desire for the object. That is to say, to judge that something is beautiful, for Kant, is different than saying that one likes something, since the latter implies an active desire that arises in connection with the feeling of the pleasure (such as saying "I like chocolate milk"); any statement implying a desire for or toward the object is a judgment of the agreeable. In that sense, aesthetic judgment is "disinterested," because it is contemplative, without the activation of desire.[9]

The second point is that while Jt are based on a subjective experience of pleasure, they also make a claim to "universality," in that they assert that everyone else who perceives the object "ought to" come to the same conclusion as they do, namely, that the object is beautiful. For Kant, when someone says they like chocolate milk,[10] they have no expectation that everyone else ought to like it as well. Connected to this point is that one cannot simply demonstrate that an object is beautiful just by referencing the concept of beauty, as one does by referencing the color green when demonstrating that a given object is green. Consequently, there are no logical or formal rules that can prove that an object is beautiful, and that can mandate universal assent to the truth of the claim. Thus, the justification for aesthetic judgment is not based on "subsumption" of the object under a *determinative* concept, which therefore renders this type of judgment *reflective*.[11] Kant's account of the mechanics of this demand for universality, and the grounding of the intersubjective validity of these judgments, will be described more fully below.

The third point is that in Jt, the subject does not presume any "end" or "purpose" through which to judge the object. In this sense, Jt are different than judgments of the good, which imply a moral framework through which to make evaluations.

The fourth point, connected to the element of "universality" (the second point outlined above), is that while one acknowledges that not everyone will make the same judgment that the object is beautiful, they "ought" to do so; this implies the concept of "necessity," which undergirds the universality of the judgment. This means that the subject feels that his experience of pleasure is a "necessary" outcome of his encounter with the object, and that therefore anyone else encountering the object should experience the same pleasure from it. Under this rubric, Kant also introduces the idea of the common sense, or "sensus communis," which he defines as a "critical faculty which in its reflective act takes account (a priori) of the mode of representation of everyone else … to weigh its judgment with the collective reason of mankind" (Kant, as quoted by Beiner, 1983, p. 50). As such, the "necessity" of the pleasure makes recourse to an expectation (or anticipation) of how others will respond to the object, which contributes to the basis for the judgment's normativity.

Returning to the mechanics of Jt, and the mechanisms for its claims to universality and necessity, we turn to Kant's notion that the pleasure of the beautiful depends on the "free play" (see Ginsborg's description, quoted below) of imagination and understanding. Kant's approach is that generally, imagination "synthesiz[es] the manifold of intuition" (Kant, quoted by Ginsborg, 2014) under the rules generated by understanding, such that sense perceptions become subsumed under concepts and are thereby rendered intelligible and accessible as cognitive percepts. However, in the experience of beauty, imagination, and understanding

> can stand in a different kind of relationship, one in which imagination's activity harmonizes with the understanding but without imagination's being constrained or governed by understanding . . . . They do this without bringing the object under any concept in particular. So rather than perceiving the object as green or square, the subject whose faculties are in free play responds to it perceptually with a state of mind which is non-conceptual, and specifically a feeling of disinterested pleasure. (Ginsborg, 2014)

That is to say, the faculty of imagination is not bound by the rule-bound schematics, or concepts, generated by the faculty of understanding, which normally guide perception and cognition. Rather, there is an interaction of "free play" between the faculties of imagination and understanding, which for Kant produces a state or feeling of a particular kind of pleasure in the subject. For Kant, this pleasure is "disinterested," in the sense that it does not necessarily imply any desire to actually possess the object.

In terms of the final step in the sequence, there is some debate as to how exactly the judgment is made, and what it in fact means to say that an object is beautiful. It would seem that the simplest approach is to say that beauty is the word,[12] or "indeterminate concept" (Ginsborg, 2014, quoting Kant), that is generated through reflection, to describe a subjective experience of a very particular kind of pleasure (the free play of the faculties). When one judges an object to be beautiful, the judgment does place this given particular (the object) under a universal, in that it can be described as belonging to the class of objects that are beautiful. That is to say, this object belongs to the class of objects that produce a particular kind of pleasure when they are subject to contemplation. However, again, this classification, or subsumption, makes use of an "indeterminate concept" (i.e., beauty); the subsumption is not determinative and cannot be demonstrated conclusively through deductions from pure logical concepts in the way that is characteristic of determinant judgments. Rather, its claims to intersubjective validity rely on claims of universality and necessity, as described above.

As such, Kant argues that universality is possible in Jt, because the same way one can expect that everyone's perceptions of an object will match their own (green, square), they can expect that the experience of regarding an object will induce in others the same interplay between the faculties (that of free play) which was engendered in them. This in turn will produce for others the same pleasure which they experienced, and will therefore prompt the same judgment of beauty.

A question can be raised, however, about the parameters of reflective judgment, as Kant's model includes the role of feeling in reflective judgment only within the context of aesthetic judgment, and only seems to refer to the affect of pleasure. We present here a series of cases, which require affect as a referent for judgment, but the emotion required is not simply one of pleasure or displeasure (although the argument can be made that they are derivatives). Additionally, these cases do in fact require the subsumption of a particular under a given universal, and do not seem dependent on the free play of the faculties, which therefore differentiates them from aesthetic judgments. Conversely, these cases are more complex and more subjective than standard determinative judgments, and also require an affective component (as the referent), which further differentiates them from cognitive and determinative judgments. Let us consider the following cases:

Consider the following judgments, are *C*'s jokes funny, or is *C* a good comedian. It would seem to be a cognitive and determinative judgment in that it is looking to subsume a particular under a given category, namely funny, or good comedian. These categories would seem to be given universals in that they do not need be generated through reflection; but at the same time, these judgments also seem to require the use of feeling as a referent, since in order to assess whether something is humorous, the judging subject would have to go through his own reactions and determine whether the feelings he had as a reaction to the jokes indicate or determine that they found them humorous. In that sense they resemble aesthetic judgments, in their subjectivity and appeal to universal assent (when someone thinks something is funny, there does seem to be an expectation that others ought to find it funny as well, which is why so often we seek to share humorous material); but of course these do not concern "beauty," and may not depend on the free play of the faculties. They also do not seem to be judgments of the agreeable, since in some sense they do seem disinterested, in that one doesn't necessarily have a desire to hear comedy, for any given reason, and can approach the question more abstractly. Additionally, they are further differentiated from judgments of the agreeable, as they seem to carry the qualities of universality and necessity, as we have mentioned.

Or consider the following questions, which seem to arise more often within the clinical context and present themselves as the type of judgments with which people who are chronically incapable of making judgments have difficulty making, and call to mind Doron et al.'s (2014) phenomenological treatment of OCD within the context of relationships: 1) Is *L* a loving person, or 2) is *L* a good babysitter? These require making use of the subjective experiences that emerge during the encounter with the other (wondering about making a commitment to L after some time spent together in a romantic relationship; making a judgment whether to trust L as a babysitter after spending a brief period observing her interactions with another child under her care) in order to make a definitive judgment that has universal (and intersubjective) validity. They rely on feeling as a referent of judgment, seemingly differentiating them from judgments of the good, but are clearly not aesthetic, and still require subsuming it under a category, such as caring, loving, and others.

The basic issue is that they are differentiated from judgments of the good in that they cannot be decided abstractly, in that they rely on components that are subjective and dependent on affective experience, which complicates any subsumption; yet, at the same time, they make a claim toward universality that goes beyond judgments of the agreeable. And, it is often these kinds of judgments with which the clinical population of compulsive doubters and those with chronic ambivalence (indecisiveness) have trouble making (should

I marry this person, is this a good place to live, is this a good school to send my children to, etc.).

In order to consider these questions more thoroughly, and to explore the degree to which Kant's model of aesthetic judgment can be applied and made relevant to the clinical context, we turn to an interesting appropriation by the political theorist Ronald Beiner (1983), who has similarly attempted to apply Kant's work on aesthetic judgment outside of the context of epistemology in order to illuminate political judgment. Beiner builds here on some initial suggestions from Hannah Arendt's late lectures (published by Beiner, 1982) on Kant's Critique of Judgment.

As a political philosopher, Beiner is most broadly concerned with an inquiry into judgment in order to restore the appropriate role of the average citizen in the political process, which in his estimation, following Habermas, has become focused, to the point of crisis, on the participation of experts and technocrats. Beiner argues that by framing judgment as a central aspect of human activity, and by demonstrating that it is not a purely subjective process but rather one that can be intersubjectively grounded, we can restore the central role of the general citizenry in the political process. Critically, Beiner argues that this intersubjective validity which is present in political judgment can hold even when those judgments are not simply applications or extensions of logical rules.

Drawing on Arendt, Beiner situates Kant's account of aesthetic judgment within this framework. He suggests that Kant is intending to address the fundamental tension inherent in aesthetic judgment, namely, the grounding of its intersubjective validity. Through what mechanisms can aesthetic judgments transcend their inherent subjectivity and the circumstances of their propagation, such that they are not only to be thought of as arbitrary and whimsical, but are sufficiently strong to make claims on others?

As Beiner outlines, Arendt is interested in developing a philosophy of political judgment, and finds in Kant's aesthetic judgment the kernel and core of her account. She is particularly interested in amplifying and making use of the concepts of taste, "enlarged mentality" and the "sensus communis" (see p. 42 for Kant's definition of this concept). Because she was interested in judgment as a capacity, she is drawn to Kant, and because she is interested in an account of the political realm, she is drawn to the intersubjective realm within which Kant situates aesthetic judgment. Ultimately, Arendt argues (as explained by Beiner, 1983, pp. 17–18) that through the "enlarged mentality," it is possible to think about a given issue from the standpoints of all mentally-represented parties (not substantively represented), which produces more valid conclusions about what should be done.

Ultimately, Beiner argues that while Kant's position as it is presented in his writings is in fact too narrow in its requirement of subsumption for all judgment, this requirement is tangential to the central elements and concerns of Kant himself in his account of reflective judgment. He reads Kant's account by marking and amplifying Kant's emphasis on the centrality of freedom and autonomy, which for Kant are engendered and maintained through the faculty of judgment as expressed through reflective judgment (and in particular, aesthetic and teleological judgments).[13] Beiner will argue that according to Kant, the central quality of judgment is that it serves as a "mediating concept between nature and freedom" (Beiner, 1983, p. 35), and that this freedom is achieved through the exercise of the imaginative and creative elements of judgments, such that they are not arrived at algorithmically and formulaically (as is the case in determinative judgments). That is to say, it is creative mental activity, unforced and undetermined, as opposed to determinative and algorithmic processing of reality, which provides the conditions for human freedom. As such, the central elements of reflective judgment can be faithfully rendered without being tethered to the issue of subsumption,[14] which therefore allows for a Kantian model of political judgment.

We begin then with Beiner's reconstruction of Kant's account of judgment, paying close attention to how the faculty of judgment as manifest in reflective judgment guarantees freedom and autonomy, and how these themes are emphasized and interwoven into Kant's model. Following our account of Beiner's reconstruction, we will then show how this account can illuminate some of the characteristics of OCD doubting that we have made as the focus for this study, including the relationship between the symptomatic behavior of OCD doubting and the more characterological construct of indecisiveness.

As mentioned, Kant distinguishes between determinant and reflective judgments, the latter, referring to aesthetic and teleological judgments. Beiner calls attention to the common point between these forms of reflective judgment, which is their notion of "finality." That is to say, in these classes of judgments we implicitly conceive of the object as if it were designed for the purpose of the reflection; either for the subject's enjoyment (in aesthetic judgments) or "to serve human purposes" (in teleological judgments) (Beiner, 1983, p. 36). This is necessary in order to establish the relevant frameworks in which the reflection will take place. For example, Beiner suggests that the study of biology requires the "idea of biological organisms as end-governed wholes, as if these objects were shaped by a rational creator in accordance with an idea of their end" (1983, p. 36). Similarly, aesthetic judgments require the notion of finality "to make it possible for us to form judgments of taste at all"[15] (Beiner, 1983, p. 36). As such, these suppositions are regulative (but not constitutive) ideas. For Beiner, these regulative ideas (which constitute the notion of finality) have serious implications for the relationship between freedom and judgment, which we will describe shortly.

Importantly, though, there is a distinction between aesthetic and teleo-logical judgments. Beiner emphasizes that for Kant, aesthetic judgments are more fundamentally subjective, in that they are defined by Kant "as the faculty of estimating formal finality (otherwise called subjective) by the feeling of pleasure or displeasure" (Kant, as quoted by Beiner, 1983). As Beiner explains, in aesthetic judgments the subject's representation is solely of the object's "form," without recourse to additional concepts or cognitive schemata through which to render the object meaningful (such as its practical function). Accordingly, the estimation of its finality (that is, the subject's ren-dering of the object and his determination about the object) is accomplished through the subject's own experience of the object (the feeling of pleasure or displeasure). Teleological judgment, however, is "the faculty of estimat-ing the real finality (objective) of nature" (Kant, as quoted by Beiner, 1983). Here, the process of reflection about nature yields the regulative supposition about "end-governed wholes" which then allows for further cognitive elabo-ration and conceptual ordering. Despite the subjectivity inherent in aesthetic judgments, Beiner notes that it is nonetheless important to bear in mind that for Kant, when we judge taste (as individual subjects) we do indeed make a claim about universality, but that in the absence of "cognitive concepts" (Beiner, 1983, p. 37) through which to determine the aesthetic quality of the object, the claim to universality is solely grounded on the "the configuration of faculties of the [judging] subject" (Beiner, 1983, p. 37). The significance of this distinction for Beiner's argument will be revisited shortly.

Beiner then proceeds to draw further attention to the elements of Kant's framework which are germane to his consideration of political judgment. Of these, we will highlight the points that are of relevance to our application of Kant's model to the clinical cases referenced earlier.

Beiner argues that for Kant, "taste is a realm of freedom" (p. 42). This is grounded in a series of observations concerning the relationship between judgment and freedom. The first concerns Kant's stipulation that judgments of beauty must be disinterested. As Beiner explains, when someone needs something (that is to say, when the subject is in a state of lacking or depriva-tion vis-à-vis the object), his evaluation of that object cannot be considered disinterested. It is by definition driven by his need, which experientially taints the capacity to judge objectively. Insofar as the object does elicit his desire, the judger will then struggle to determine objectively whether the object should in fact be desired, and cannot make a disinterested assessment of its quality. Accordingly, if one desires a given object, his assessment that this object is beautiful may also simply be a reflection of his desire for it. As such, judgments of taste (aesthetic judgment) can only be considered distinct from judgments of the agreeable (and can only truly be made) when the subject is not in a state of deprivation vis-à-vis the object. Critically, for Beiner, this point is not only technical, but also thematic; the capacity to engage in aesthetic judgment implies a state of being in which man is not contingent upon nature (its contingencies and dictates), but rather can stand outside of it, in a state of freedom.

Beiner makes an additional observation here as well, in connection to the relationship between imagination and freedom. He suggests that for Kant, aesthetic judgment is "free judgment" (Beiner, 1983, p. 43) due to the imagination, which "entertains the mind in a free activity" (Beiner, 1983, quoting Kant, p. 42). In this context, Beiner adduces Kant's characterization of art as similar to play. Through its openness and spontaneity, it is the imagination which creates the environment for the particular qualities of mentation necessary for aesthetic judgment. We will return shortly to discuss Beiner's expansion of this point.

Beiner continues to highlight the relationship between judgment and freedom by drawing on Kant's notion of finality. As we have mentioned, Beiner notes the distinction between aesthetic and teleological judgment with regards to the notion of finality; that in teleological judgment, the judgment pertains to the objective finality of the object (though grounded in a regulative notion of finality, as explained above) and its ultimate purpose. However, in aesthetic judgment, the judgment pertains only to the formal finality of the object. The quality of beauty is not an objective quality which inheres in the object independently of the observing subject. Rather, it can only be assessed through consideration of the subject's experience of the object.

In Beiner's reading of Kant, this contrast sets up a tension between two different ways of representing and experiencing the world. The notions of "ends" and objective finality (which are determined in teleological judgments) imply necessity, which entail the foreclosure of possibility and choice. The essence of teleological judgment is a perception of nature as it must be, by necessity; and this in turn leads to judgments which are grounded "upon heteronomy" (Beiner, 1983, quoting Kant, p. 47), as the judging subject arrives at a determination about why things are the way they are. In aesthetic judgment, however, the subject's cognitive faculties are receptive to "free play," driven by imagination and not fully constrained by the understanding. It is therefore a freer subjective experience than teleologically oriented perception, and one that is grounded in "autonomy."

As such, teleology must remain distinct from aesthetics; the teleological perspective represents a threat to freedom and autonomy, because it gives rise to a linear and programmatic mode of thought which limits the imaginative mode of thinking and the undetermined potentialities which might emerge therefrom. Beiner argues that this distinction, and its implications for the relationship between judgment and freedom, is central to Kant's model of aesthetic judgment, and is thematically connected to Kant's larger consideration of "freedom as against nature" (Beiner, p. 47).

Notwithstanding the differences noted above between aesthetic and teleological judgments, Beiner argues that imagination is critical for both forms of judgment, and is central to Kant's model of judgment as a whole. He argues that in teleological judgment, it is the imagination which allows for positing of ideas about the objective finality of nature and natural phenomena, without which one could not "transcend the given particulars" accessible through sensory perception. Importantly, within this context, Beiner suggests that the essence of judgment (in all its forms) is "to rise above particulars as given in sensory perception in order to subsume them under a universal" (p. 49). This formulation of judgment as the "transcending of particulars" will become critical for our discussion at the end of this chapter.

Next, Beiner takes up a consideration of the common sense, or the "sensus communis," and the role it plays in Kant's model. For Kant, the qualifications of necessity and universality inherent in judgments of taste (the belief that everyone else who perceives the object must also experience it as pleasurable) are grounded in common sense, which carries for Kant a particular definition:

> a critical faculty which in its reflective act takes account (a priori) of the mode of representation of everyone else, as it were, to weigh its judgment with the collective reason of mankind. (Kant, quoted by Beiner, p. 50)

As Beiner explains, the sensus communis is "not . . . some external sense" (Kant, quoted by Beiner, p. 49) alien to the subject's own mentation and cognition. It is also not a constitutive referent of actual opinions. Rather, it means "weighing the judgment, not so much with actual, as rather with merely possible, judgments of others, and by putting ourselves in the position of everyone else" (Kant, quoted by Beiner, p. 51).

Within the faculties of cognition, then, is a capacity to anticipate and to formulate expectations of how the collective of "others" would see and judge the object. This ability to think from the perspective of this collective other and make use of these expectations is used during the process of making judgments of taste as a scaffolding guide for our own judgments. The result is an "enlarged mentality" (Kant, quoted by Beiner, p. 51) and the ability to transcend the "subjective conditions" (Kant, quoted by Beiner, p. 51) that would otherwise bias one's judgments. This point has implications for the intersubjective validity of aesthetic judgments, as will emerge shortly.

For Beiner (and here he follows Arendt's earlier suggestions), the role of common sense has significant implications for political judgment, because it means that judgment is public. This is true in two senses. First, judgments use the public (as a collective) as a referent. And second, they appeal to valid-ity from the collective, in the form of public assent and agreement. As such, judgment can be understood as a public act taking place within the public (and therefore, political) realm.

This point is critical for our consideration as well because it poses an important question. If, through the "enlarged mentality," judgments rely on the incorporation of an external (though disembodied) voice, why do they (assuming that they do) feel as if they are our own, and in what sense are they are own? To transpose the question to a psychological framework, it is almost as if Kant is describing an additional psychical object within the mind that weighs in on judgments, in that it is used as a referent for judg-ment. Is this voice experienced as self-alien, as other? Or is it experienced as "purely self" (or the authentic self), such that the judgment that incorporates it is experienced as deriving from the self, and not externally compelled? Additionally, how are we to understand the development of the "enlarged mentality"? Even within the realm of aesthetic judgments, Kant's account of the sensus communis raises a question surrounding the degree to which this sense may be cultivated and shaped by exposure to the judgments of oth-ers. Kant seems to take the presence of the "sensus communis" as a given, and Arendt seems to indicate that there are those whose capacities to make use of the "enlarged mentality" are more or less developed, but how does it develop, and how might we account for it psychologically? For Kant the issue of self vs. other is addressed philosophically; the enlarged mind frees the subject of bias and prejudice, and allows for greater objectivity, which is the truest form of freedom from nature. However, the tension inherent in the objectivity of the "sensus communis" between authentic self-experience as opposed to acquiescence to a self-alien perspective still needs to be resolved psychologically. To address this fundamental question, we will later make use in subsequent chapters of object-relations theory, the development of the superego, the nature of identification and internalization, and look at the writ-ings of Winnicott and Vygotsky's treatment of inner talk.

We return now to Beiner's consideration of Kant's model of reflective judgment. He argues that Kant is aware of the complexity of aesthetic judgment, and acknowledges that "correct subsumption of particulars in reflective judgment . . . is much more problematical than the rendering of a logical judgment" (Beiner, p. 53), but that the difficulty of the task does not negate the paradigm of subsumption. How then, does the subsumption happen? As Beiner explains, for Kant, the nature of the subsumption is such that it depends on the distinction between "contention" and "dispute." Dispute entails "decision by means of proofs" (Beiner, 1983, p. 53), such that the demand for assent is made through logical procession from definite concepts, which compel agreement through their logical force. In aesthetic judgment, there can be no definitive resolution established through sheer logic. Nonetheless, "contentions" about taste and beauty are both possible and warranted, where one hopes to convince another of the rightness of their position while acknowledging that it cannot be compelled. Importantly, Beiner again underscores that contentions about taste are not purely arbitrary, and do "depend upon a concept" (Kant, quoted by Beiner, p. 54); that is to say, judgments of taste do derive from the indeterminate concept of beauty, though they cannot be logically demonstrated as necessarily deriving from the concept. In this reading of Kant, Beiner emphasizes that the "enlarged reference" is the grounding upon which judgments of taste can be intersubjectively valid, in that we make such judgments with the collective in mind, and therefore can legitimately hope for universal assent.

Within this discussion about the "sensus communis," Beiner again revisits the tension he has previously highlighted between autonomy and heteronomy and Kant's sensitivity to this tension. He notes that Kant acknowledges that incorporating the viewpoints of others into one's own judgment risks the potential for undermining the autonomy of judgment. Importantly, he suggests that for Kant, this form of heteronomy also limits the responsibility of the judging subject. As we will explain, the connection between autonomy and responsibility is central to Beiner's formulation of reflective judgment.

Having laid out some of the central pieces of Beiner's rendering of Kant, we turn now to his critique of Kant's model, and then to his own formulation of reflective judgment. Beiner will argue that in order for the essential elements of Kant's model of reflective judgment to hold, the category of reflective judgments must be broadened outward, and the distinction between affective and cognitive judgments must be eased.[16] His position here will allow us to make use of Kantian models of judgment in order to explicate clinical phenomena. We first lay out the components of his argument.

Beiner argues that by the very nature of Kant's enterprise (composing the Critique of Judgment), it is implied that the formula of subsumption itself is insufficient to provide a full account of judgment. Otherwise, he could simply have defined judgment as the subsumption of a particular under a universal, and stopped there. Rather, according to Beiner, Kant acknowledges that "straightforward subsumption" (Beiner, 1983, p. 109) is not possible in aesthetic judgment, and instead attempts to describe the process of a more "problematical subsumption" (Beiner, 1983, p. 109) where the universal is more "elusive" (Beiner, 1983, p. 112) and its relationship to the particular is more ambiguous. As Beiner explains, it is this kind of "problematical" subsumption which is operative in aesthetic judgment.

In this distinction between "straightforward" and "problematical" subsumption, the former is essentially algorithmic and formulaic in nature; there is some predetermined outcome that one is to arrive at through following a given train of thought. Beiner argues that this kind of subsumption is in tension with the notion of autonomy (see our discussion in note 13, below); as mentioned above, he maintains that it is a condition of autonomy that the judging subject bear responsibility for their judgment, and algorithmic reasoning of this sort removes responsibility and accountability from the judging subject since they were merely following a set of logical rules to arrive at the correct decision. Moreover, it also infringes on the "right" (Beiner, 1983, p. 112) of the judging subject to form his own independent judgments. As such, Beiner maintains that in order for Kant's account to appropriately center the notion of autonomy within aesthetic judgment, it must also deemphasize the "neatness" (see the below quote from Beiner) and linearity of the subsumption. As Beiner explains,

> the weighing of given particulars and their careful adjustment to the demands of an elusive universal—a universal under which the particular cannot be neatly subsumed—are, then, the matters of the responsibility of the judging subject . . . the individual judging subject cannot be deprived of his right to personal judgment by some objectively determinable universal rule. (Beiner, 1983, p. 112)

Beiner further seeks to emphasize the notion of autonomy within judgment, and proceeds thusly to critique the "overly rigid dichotomization of the cognitive and non-cognitive" (p. 113) in Kant's model. He notes that even for cognitive judgments, which Kant would consider determinative, there are often elements that are "reflective," in that the subsumption is problematical and complex, and requires the "discretion" of the judging subject (we will shortly discuss Beiner's examples for these kinds of judgments). A strict reading of Kant would not allow for the place of discretion within determinative judgments, and would not generally acknowledge problematical subsumption within the class of determinative judgments, since typically subsumptions must derive directly from concepts and are subject to formal logic. However, Beiner argues that if we are to take seriously the connection between judgment and autonomy, then the notion of "discretion" must somehow become accommodated even within the rubric of determinative judgments. Without this, the creative elements involved in these kinds of judgments, which require the imagination and discretion of the judging subject, remain unaccounted for. As such, Beiner moves to the position that the relationship between determinative and reflective judgments is more complex than it would seem from a simple reading of Kant.

Consequently, Beiner reaches a new, more expansive, definition for reflective judgment:

> Reflective judgment is necessarily problematical subsumption of the particulars under an elusive universal. This always implies a logical gap between what is

available for judging and what is required in the way of judgment, and it falls to the human responsibility if the judging subject is to bridge this gap. (Beiner, 1983, p. 114)

Beiner's formulation of reflective judgment and his position about the complexities even within determinative judgments are critical for our discussion; they open a path to expand Kant's model to the cases that are germane to the clinical setting, and to our consideration of compulsive doubting.

Before returning to the cases we introduced earlier, we first lay out Beiner's consideration of cases which are cognitive and straightforwardly determinative judgments according to Kant, but with his expanded definition of reflective judgment he can now consider from within the framework of Kantian reflective judgment. While his goal is to build up to a consideration of political judgment from within this rubric, it is not necessary for our purposes to pursue his full account of political judgment, but to appropriate his emendations to Kant's basic distinction between cognitive and affective judgments.

Beiner intends to delineate the parameters of political judgments, and by doing so reconsiders, under his expanded definition of reflective judgment, different kinds of (hitherto) cognitive judgments for their reflective elements. He considers first the class of practical judgments, and discusses the example of a chess game. The determination of what is the best move is cognitive, and in theory, should be classified as determinative, in that it follows from clear rules and objectives inherent in the game's structure. However, it is often difficult to choose from among a range of credible and compelling options and strategies, which move is actually the best one. As Beiner argues:

> even where the exact rules or algorithms are available, meta rules are not available for application of the first-order rules—so that first-order judgment is determinant, second-order judgment, reflective . . . what is determinant at one level can be reflective at another level. (1983, p. 131)

Rather, where the correct and appropriate application cannot readily be made, a relatively subjective determination must be made, in that it cannot be arrived at purely from a computational sense.[17] Nonetheless, the player feels that he has made "the right move," and as such, there is an appeal to universal assent. The "various features of the situation that justify one's choice" (Biener, 1983, p. 132) of a move point to an intersubjective validity, in that rationality is operative, and the correctness of the move is subject to contention. Additionally, Beiner highlights another reflective element that is operative in chess, which is that imagination is at play, so to speak. The range of possible moves has to be "conjured," as well as the likely responses of one's opponent (which, it might be added, can involve a consideration of their skill level or playing tendencies; are they aggressive or conservative, etc.).

Beiner then goes on to consider judgments of character. He argues that in order to consider the quality of another person's integrity or honesty, one must base this judgment on "an implicit claim about one's own personal qualities, such as reliability and trustworthiness" (1983, p. 136). While these claims about ourselves cannot be proven in a formal sense, they "point to the qualities of insight, maturity, experience, objectivity, and so on, which ground and give weight to judgment" (1983, p. 136) and form the basis upon which others are willing to rely on the assessment of the judging subject. As such, the judging subject makes the following argument for universality: "if I judge a person to be unsavory, you are likely to be inclined to judge likewise . . . trust me, for my judgments have proven accurate in the past, and if my judgment fails me here I risk the diminution of whatever credibility I now enjoy" (1983, p. 136). As such, there is also an assumption of responsibility inherent in this judgment, since it implicitly invites others (as described in the argument for universality) to rely on the assessment of the judging subject.

At this point, it is appropriate to revisit our question concerning the determination of the loving babysitter. We have framed the question differently, not basing it as much on an implicit claim of the judger's reliability, but grounding it in the subjective experience of seeing the babysitter interact with a child. We argue here that according to Beiner, this example should be classified as a reflective judgment. First, as Beiner articulates in the chess example, it requires the operation of imagination, in order to conjure what it would be like to be the child. Secondly, it relies on a feeling that is inter-subjectively valid, in that the observer could point to various behaviors and patterns of behavior and make plausible and justifiable attributions about the caregiver's intentions, as well as their overall degree of attunement and attention to the child's needs. Facial expressions and tone of voice could also be used to look at levels of affection and aggression, or indifference, for that matter. As such, reason is operative, as are the conceptual categories of good, empathic, caring, and so on. However, while these concepts are active, their application to the situation is not clearly delineated. There are likely to be conflicting or ambivalent reactions, interpretations, and attributions, thereby making a straightforward subsumption difficult, and requiring a "bridging of the gap" in the search for a problematical subsumption under an elusive universal. Additionally, this judgment of the babysitter implies an assumption of responsibility, since the consequences for the leaving of one's child under the babysitter's care rest solely on the judgment of the observer.

Thus, we can conclude that Kant's model of reflective judgment, particularly as it has been expanded in Beiner's formulation, is a fruitful approach for a consideration of the clinical phenomena present in compulsive doubting.

At this point, then, it is appropriate to restate a few points about the relation-ship between OCD doubting and the faculty of judgment, and thereby tie together and clarify some of the points and connections we have suggested in this chapter.

First, more broadly, Beiner's notion of "problematic subsumption" affords us ground to suggest that a persistent and pervasive inability to arrive at conclusions and make determinations itself reflects an element of pathology of the self, independent of the subjective distress that often accompanies the agonies of indecision and ambivalence. Additionally, it also suggests that this pattern is reflective of pathology even when manifest in situations that are inherently ambiguous, such as within the context of romantic relationships. It is true that in such situations, uncertainty and ambivalence are often war-ranted; it might be argued that the uncertainty and ambivalence are warranted even if they produce significant distress. However, Beiner's rendering of Kant's model points us to (and strengthens) a critical distinction between the constructs of IU (intolerance of uncertainty) and indecisiveness (as a persis-tent difficulty with making decisions themselves). The justification for both of these points is that for Beiner, reflective judgment is at its core the ability to make judgments specifically if they *are* complex and problematical. In Beiner's reading of Kant, the ability to make an ultimate determination about something, either an internal state or an external circumstance, and generate a unified apperception (*Ich denke*) in propositional (and therefore definitive) form is a central faculty of the mind, and a core element of human freedom. The diminishment of this faculty therefore means that a given person (whose capacity to judge is diminished) is less free and less autonomous (that is, in the experiential sense), which can readily be understood as an indication of pathology of the self. As we have explained, this diminishment is meaningful even in the absence of significant distress, and even in conditions of inherent ambiguity.

This leads to the next point, which is that Beiner's rendering of Kantian judgment allows us to strengthen the conceptual link between the two types of uncertainty that we outlined in the introduction: the uncertainty present in relatively "determinative" classical doubting compulsions, such as repeat-edly checking that the door is locked, and the uncertainties that require more "problematical subsumptions," such as those within the context of romantic relationships. We can say that according to Beiner, they are related in two ways. First, both require a determination to be made about something, and the arrival at some definite conclusion (either simple or complex); in the words of Beiner that we cited above, "to rise above particulars as given in sensory perception." As such, they can both be said to reflect impairments in the capacity to judge. Second, they often entail the element of responsibil-ity, either for the safety of those inside the house, or for the gravity of the choice to commit to their partner. For Beiner, judgment itself requires that the subject assumes and accepts the responsibility for the consequences of the determination, and this assumption of responsibility is central to his definition of reflective judgment. We can therefore connect these two typologies of OCD doubting to the concept of responsibility, reflecting the observations referenced in the introduction about "inflated responsibility" and its role within OCD; patients with OCD experience the responsibility for making these determinations to be overwhelming. Furthermore, we can now conceptualize the experience of overwhelming responsibility about judgments as an extension of a diminished capacity for judgment, and not merely as an affective byproduct.

Last, as we have noted, Beiner's formulation of an expanded Kantian account of reflective judgment, with its definition of "the subsumption of problematical particulars under an elusive universal" and its emphasis on the "enlarged mentality" raises psychological questions about the internalization of "universals," and the degree to which this internalization is experienced as authentic to the self or as self-alien. We thus turn our attention to the psychological treatment of "internalization," beginning with psychoanalytic conceptualizations of superego formation and internalization. We will begin with a presentation of Schafer's (1968/1990) thorough overview and treatment of these subjects.

NOTES

1. This account draws primarily from the Stanford Encyclopedia of Philosophy entry "Kant's Theory of Judgment," authored by Robert Hanna (2017) which provides a thorough and concise overview.

2. For the specific definition of a faculty, see Hanna (2017).

3. In this sense, then, Kant prefigures some of the central elements of the contemporary account of cognition as represented in the computational model of cognition, in that cognition is not just content based, but also procedural, and unfolds according to latent schemata.

4. As noted by Hanna (2017), there is significant debate and ambiguity in Kant concerning whether imagination is part of sensibility, or is an autonomous faculty. For our purposes, it is sufficient merely to note its function and characteristics.

5. Note that for Winnicott, infants do indeed have a concept of time, which he refers to as "x+y+z time" (1971). While not critical for our discussion here, we will return to this point more fully in our discussion of Winnicott in chapter 6.

6. This account draws primarily from Hanna Ginsborg's (2014) entry in the Stanford Encyclopedia of Philosophy, "Kant's Aesthetics and Teleology."

7. In this chapter, we retain the Kantian term "subsumption," due to its centrality and importance within the philosophical literature, as well as its particular and specific technical connotations.

8. Again, our outline here follows Ginsborg's account. This point will be explored more fully in our discussion below (see below note 16).

9. While the precise connection between beauty and pleasure is exceedingly complex within Kant's system (see Ginsborg, 2014 for a fuller treatment of this issue), it can be said that while the determination that something is beautiful might lead to desire for the object, that is not the source of the judgment, nor is it a necessary outcome. One can find a painting in a museum to be beautiful knowing full well the impossibility of ever attaining it.

10. Importantly, for Kant, judgments of the agreeable are distinguished from value judgments, whether they are aesthetic or moral. Value judgments that are fundamentally moral or normative, what Kant terms "judgments of the good," are eminently not disinterested. While clearly of importance, they are tangential to our discussion because for Kant they must be grounded in universal laws and are not reflective judgments.

11. In fact, Kant is somewhat ambiguous as to whether beauty is in fact a "concept of the object," and whether there is any subsumption under the concept beauty at all (see Ginsborg, 2014). We will work with the assumption that the judgment itself is a subsumption under the "indeterminate concept" of beauty (again following one of the approaches described by Ginsborg, 2014), but that this subsumption is not the justification for its universality and necessity. We will address this point again further in the course of our outline.

12. As noted earlier, this follows one of the possibilities mentioned by Ginsborg in her presentation of this issue.

13. It should be noted that, for Kant, the concepts of freedom and autonomy are essentially connected to the issues of free will and moral choice. That is, Kant maintains that man does have free will and moral choice. As such, this notion of freedom stands in contrast to the determinism which for Kant isinherent in the epistemological framework that structures an understanding of nature. However it is important for our argument to note that Beiner's discussion of autonomy in the present context is situated within Kant's framework of reflective judgment and is distinct from Kant's treatment of morality and ethics.

14. As we will see, Beiner differentiates between *purely* determinative subsumption, which he refers to as "straightforward subsumption," and "problematical subsumption," which he proposes as the general process operative in both aesthetic judgments as well as the many instances in which judgment (even cognitive judgments) cannot be understood as purely determinative. It is this distinction which is crucial for our discussion.

15. Seemingly, this means as follows: in order to make a judgment about taste, there must be a subsumption under the indeterminate concept of "beauty." Accordingly, in order to determine (by reflecting on one's experience of the object, as outlined above) whether a given object should be subsumed under the indeterminate concept of beauty, this requires the supposition that the category of beauty (and the concomitant appraisal of the degree to which the object can be meaningfully subsumed under this category) is relevant to the object. That is to say, a work of art prompts us to judge whether it is beautiful (if we suppose that it was intended in fact

to be beautiful) whereas, for example, a box of nails positioned next to a hammer does not prompt us to consider that it may have been an artistic arrangement and does not raise at all the question about whether this arrangement is beautiful or not.

16. This essential position is also maintained by the Kant scholars Longuenesse (2003) and Allison (2001) in their treatment of reflective judgment (though they differ in significant ways, these are beyond the scope of our discussion). We cite here Longuenesse's (2003) summary of their position:

"In clarifying the latter—the reflective judgment—Allison refers to the analyses I have proposed, in Kant and the Capacity to Judge, of the role of reflection in Kant's theory of judgment in the first Critique. He agrees with me that in empirical knowledge, all determinative judgments must have a reflective component: even if we have available to us the relevant concepts under which to subsume individual objects, there is always an initial stage at which we apprehend what is given to our senses and grope, as it were, for the relevant concept." (p. 145)

17. Beiner's book was written in 1983; since then, computers have been programmed to play chess at the highest levels, something which Beiner did not consider possible; nonetheless, his point stands as an example.

Chapter 2

Internalization and Superego Development

Contours of the Self

Up to this point, we have proposed the following framework through which to approach the conceptual and clinical issues within the symptomology of compulsive doubting: We began with Dar's (2000) work highlighting the distinction between cognitive and affective elements of "knowing" which emerged from a study demonstrating lower levels of confidence in OC checkers compared to healthy controls even relative to actual performance. We then discussed Lazarov et al.'s (2010) model of Seeking Proxies, which maintains that OCD patients rely on external referents to determine internal states. We next added the ROCD framework (Doron et al., 2014), which develops the particular clusters of obsessive thoughts, preoccupations, and doubts which often occur within relationships. Last, we included research suggesting the phenomenon of trait-level indecisiveness. Tying together these four strands, we have taken the position that OCD doubting reflects a broader, more global difficulty with decision-making, above and beyond metacognitive factors. We have proposed that these difficulties pertain to a more fundamental psychical capacity, that of making determinations and rendering judgments. Our focus has been to suggest that a broader Kantian framework for judgment as a distinct faculty of mind best accounts for the issues which we raised.

We now transition to a consideration of the viability of transposing this expanded Kantian framework of reflective judgment into a broader psychological account. To do so, we will propose that Kant's more static and transcendental[1] model of judgment can be grounded within the trajectory of psychological development. To clarify further, we are not addressing here the development of the actual **capacity** to judge; rather, we will suggest that the subject's attitudes and beliefs about exercising this capacity are critically important, and emerge from within the trajectory of psychological development. Accordingly, we will consider the role of psychological development in the internalization and development of the sensus communis as well the acquisition of some normative concepts required for making judgments. Following our thoughts in the preceding section, we can restate three points critical for a psychological account of Kantian judgment: 1) if judgment is the subsumption of the particular under the universal, how does the subject acquire, to begin with, the requisite categories to make the kinds of normative judgments we discussed in the previous chapter? 2) How, developmentally, does one achieve the capacity for the "enlarged mentality" of the sensus communis? 3) What allows for the subject to experience, as his own, judgments which incorporate the sensus communis? Kant's account is transcendental; he implicitly assumes the presence of mature and developed mental processes, and does not concern himself with questions of their development.

As we noted at the conclusion of the previous section, a consideration of these issues seems to revolve around the psychological process of internalization. We will present a broad account of internalization drawing first from the work of Schafer that dwells in the realm of psychoanalytic theory, and then move to the theories of Mead and Vygotsky.

Schafer's (1968/1990) analysis, in particular, of the processes involved in internalization provides us with the tools and language to more precisely articulate the object-relational dynamics at play in the process of judgment, and especially the dialectics between the self-alien and self-congruent elements of the external world which come in to play in the process of judgment. We begin then with an overview of Schafer's analysis, paying particular attention to how his articulation of the processes at play during internalization emerge within the development of the superego,[2] which will become central to our discussion of object-relations and judgment.

For Schafer, the key to clarifying the concept of internalization lies in elucidating the distinction between two processes, that of identification, and that of introjection. The thrust of Schafer's endeavor is to delineate the precise characteristics and dynamics of each of these processes, and by doing so, arrive as well at a more nuanced and precise definition of the basic mechanics and contours of the psychological self. We will provide here an overview of Schafer's project, which will in turn provide us with an important framework through which to consider the questions rose in the previous chapter.

Schafer orients his account of internalization by noting its centrality to the broad framework of psychoanalytic theory. However, as Schafer notes, the processes involved in internalization have often been referred to by other terms (such as identification, introjection, and incorporation) in an "uncoordinated, often implicit variety of ways" (p. 4), and therefore, arriving at a precise metapsychological definition of internalization has been elusive. In response, Schafer's intends to provide a more systematic analysis of the various dynamics and processes of internalization. His account focuses particular attention upon the concepts of introjection and identification, which he deems as central to the broader framework of internalization.

Schafer traces the emergence of the concept of internalization within the psychoanalytic literature, beginning with Freud, and then focusing on Hartmann. According to Schafer (p. 8), Freud's most explicit description of the process of internalization comes in a late formulation of superego function:

> A portion of the external world has, at least partially, been abandoned as an object and has instead, by identification, been taken into the ego and thus become an integral part of the inner world. This new psychical agency continues to carry on the functions which have hitherto been performed by people in the external world. (Freud, 1938, as cited by Schafer)

Schafer then introduces two definitions of internalization proposed by Hartmann; the first in 1939, and the second, proposed jointly with Loewenstein, in 1962. In his earlier definition, Hartmann seeks to situate internalization within a developmental framework that allows for a strong focus on the role that signal anxiety plays in the emergence of thought:

> an increased independence of the organism from the environment, so that *reactions* (italics mine) which originally occurred in relation to the external world are increasingly displaced into the interior of the organism.[3] (1939, cited by Schafer, p. 8)

In his subsequent definition, Hartmann proposes that "we would speak of internalization when *regulations* (italics added) that have taken place in interaction with the outside world are replaced by inner regulations."

Here, Hartmann substitutes the word *regulation* for *reaction*, which to Schafer's understanding is a significant development and advancement in conceptualization, and reflects a desire to situate the process of internalization within the "matrix of object relationships" (p. 8). Schafer understands that Hartmann is attempting to get at the internalization of something that transcends mere information and praxis (what to do and what not to do, meaning, a schematic structure). That is to say, in Hartmann's earlier definition, it is really only *information* that is "taken in"; from being told by others and by observing others, one learns the proper interpretation of various stimuli present in the external world, and the appropriate reactions to them. The mind, as the intellectual apparatus which carries out these interpretations and initiates reactions, develops as a part of this learning process, and eventually enables one to simulate and think through on one's own the range of potential environmental stimuli and potential outcomes and reactions, without needing to consult with parents and other authorities.

However, in Hartmann's second definition, the term suggests to Schafer that what is taken in is not merely abstract schematic information, what to do or what not to do. Rather, it is suggestive of motivation as well, which is superordinate to the behavioral schematics (p. 11). This is an important point and one to which we shall return when outlining Schafer's own proposed definition of internalization. Moreover, Schafer's explication of the term "regulation" will be critical for our consideration of the trajectory of internalization and superego development within the framework of compulsive doubting.

Because Hartmann's definition does not address the distinction between more specific types of internalization, and does not distinguish between introjection and identification, Schafer finds that his definition is incomplete, and a more precise formulation is needed. Building on his understanding of the central points of Hartmann's definition, Schafer proposes his own formulation as follows:

> Internalization refers to all those processes by which the subject transforms real or imagined regulatory interactions with his environment, and real or imagined characteristics of his environment, into inner regulations and characteristics. (p. 9)

While Schafer's style is exegetical, presenting a broad definition and then circling back to unpack each phrase, we will try to highlight some of the essential points that are needed for our account and relevant to our path of inquiry.

Returning again to Schafer's definition, we provide here his explanation for the word "inner," which importantly provides a clearer explanation for the referents of inner vs outer in the psychological field:

> Inner indicates that the subject locates the previously external regulatory agent within some self-boundary. (p. 10)

Later in his discussion, Schafer identifies three ways a subject conceives of such self-boundaries, and how one understands the boundary between self and other, inside and outside. These include self-as-place, self-as-object, and self-as-agent. We will revisit the precise definitions of these terms as our discussion proceeds.

Regarding the term "regulation," Schafer here wants to maintain the focus on the dialogical elements of the interaction between the subject and his environment, as well as the ways that they transcend merely schematic sequences of behavior. Importantly, as we will see, Schafer emphasizes the centrality of motivation within his discussion of regulatory interactions, and argues that it is the motivation of the regulation, and not just its function, which becomes internalized. For Schafer, it is ultimately the framework of motivation which provides the language to appropriately render the metapsychological nature of psychical structures, such as ego and superego, and processes, such as defenses. And thus, for Schafer, the superego too is best understood as a system of "regulatory motives" (p. 13) which guide behavior.

For example, if we are talking about a regulatory interaction with an external object, we might say that a parent is demanding that the child behave, or demanding a certain kind of behavior in a certain kind of situation. To say then that this regulation has become internalized, we would be saying that the child now experiences this same demand in the given situation, in the absence (or independently) of the actual demanding parent. The ultimate behavioral response to that demand (now internal), which is acquiescence and compliance, is now initiated by the child themselves, without the coercive elements and contingencies created by the parents. As such, Schafer argues that we are now talking about a process through which external *motivations* have become taken in, so that they are now (at least to some extent) experienced as arising from inside (and from the self), rather than out (from an external environmental pressure), and have created a change in the subject's motivational structure; something that he previously did not want to do or acquiesce to has now become something which he feels to be internally necessary and compelled (and perhaps even worthwhile) to do.[4]

We conclude this section of our overview of Schafer's treatment of internalization by noting that for Schafer, the process of internalization is really dimensional, and not binary; some external regulations may become more clearly "stamped by self-representations" (p. 15) than others, and the extent to which some motivations may have been internalized may be more tenuous or context-dependent than others, resulting in either more or less "stability" (p. 15) for any given internalization.

Having laid out what constitutes internalization itself, namely the transformation of externally indexed matter (including regulations, characteristics, or objects) into the self-boundary, Schafer now sets out to describe the particular characteristics of two central "internalizing processes" (p. 15), those of identification and introjection.

For Schafer, the process of identification is the process of modifying "motives and behavior patterns, and the self-representations corresponding to them" (p. 140) "in order to increase one's resemblance to an object taken as a model" (p. 16). This resemblance can include desires of "being like, the same as, and merged with one or more representations of that object" (p. 140), depending on the level of organization and process. If the identification takes place at the level of primary process (which seeks merger, incorporation, and works within a more fluid boundary between self and other), identifications involve changes in self-representation driven by magical thinking and primary process. At the level of secondary process, which recognizes a firm distinction between self and other, identifications are governed more appropriately by "being like," and often involve "deliberate imitation and learning" (p. 151). Typically, identifications reflect a "wish to experience as his own something he has hitherto found in the other person" (p. 156). Importantly, Schafer notes that identifications derive from, act upon, and are mediated by the subject's object-representations of the other person, and not with their actuality; these representations are themselves derived from the ways the subject has come to experience the other person and the various meanings and interpretations he has supplied to make sense of their interactions.

As Shafer argues, identifications cannot really be understood as a development of new psychical capacities. Rather, "they involve selective reorganization of already existing wishes, behavior patterns, capacities, viewpoints, emphases—and quite possibly earlier identifications too" (p. 147). Indeed, it is the "selective reorganization" of wishes, and "transformed pleasure-pain possibilities" (p. 147) that constitute the core of this process.[5]

Here, Schafer draws heavily on his earlier exposition of motivation, in which internalization is a process of motivational realignment. He provides the illustration of superego development, and in his example describes how a child's superego development leads to "a selective reorganization" (p. 147) of goals and motives, "strategies of restraint and renunciation" (p. 148), and to shifts in the nature of the child's self-representations. Ultimately, this transformation is profound, and the internalization so thorough, that the child's adherence and commitment to the moral code is not manifestly tethered to or influenced by any ongoing conflict or the vicissitudes of the relationship with the parent. The internalized system of regulatory motives has now acquired "autonomy" (p. 177) from the original identification. As Schafer puts it, it is not meaningful to describe a "man's moral code" (p. 177) as an actual identification with his father. Though the superego is derived from a child's identification with his father, through the "selective reorganization" (p. 147) of the child's wishes, motives, and self-representations, the superego is no longer merely an identification; it has instead become an "autonomous, integrated, and stable component" (p. 177) of the child's personality. This, for Schafer, is the process through which the superego is instantiated within the "subjective self" (p. 178) as moral code and conscience.[6]

There is an additional point which we note here, and will return to as well. Though generally speaking, the superego becomes integrated into the subjective self, at times the superego can also feel external and self-alien. This is particularly apparent within the phenomenon of self-criticism, which implies that "one part of the self is criticizing another" (p. 18). The resolution of this issue will wait until our sketch of Schafer's conceptualization of introjects.

Schafer also proposes to address the underlying question of identification; what fuels the process of identification to begin with?[7] While conceding that the motivations for any given identification may involve an almost endless array of heterogeneous and idiosyncratic needs and wishes vis-à-vis the object, he proposes five main lenses through which to analyze motivation within the context of identification: content, genetic level, complexity, conceptual level, and point of view.

Content refers to any "particular libidinal wish or an aggressive wish" (p. 163). Genetic level refers to stages in development, such as Oedipal or pre-oedipal. An identification may be fueled by more than one wish, and may be associated with more than one genetic level, which is captured by the term complexity. Some wishes are more concrete, such as a desire to be fed, and others are more abstract, such as a desire to be taken care of. These should be mapped out by their conceptual level. And last, each motive can be examined through a given point of view; namely, how it relates to the structure of psychic organization; whether it represents an ego defense or a libidinal gratification, whether it moves the subject closer to integration and individuation, or whether it is regressive and moves him closer to fracture and helplessness.

As such, for Schafer, the essential model of identification that emerges is as follows: identification is the process through which some quality or entity in the external world is "taken in." This process of taking in involves a desire and a belief, implicit and explicit, that the quality is attainable through the process of becoming similar to the person bearing the quality (imitation). This is the implicit logic of identification. Consequently, the process of identification involves a change in the self; a person's "attitudes and motivations" change, in the sense that his motivational structure becomes reoriented either toward a different goal, or becomes remodeled (and therefore modified) after the perceived tendencies and patterns of the object of identification.

Thus, for example, a child who is rebellious but has begun to identify with his father, perceived by the child to be a man of upstanding character of high integrity, would experience a change in his motivational structure. His destructive impulses might recede, while his desires to adhere to the same quality of moral code, to emulate discipline (perhaps as a proxy for strength, or a way of attaining the respect accorded to the father) and integrity, might emerge. Additionally, he might desire further emotional closeness to the father, and would therefore experience new desires and impulses that would occasion the closeness, while impulses that threaten the closeness might recede, as well as become coded as aversive, threatening or dangerous.

Since all these desires emerge from within the motivational structure, and the terminal-point for the identification itself is the self, the outcome of a successful identification is that the assimilated elements become experienced as contiguous and consonant with the self. In fact, if the process of identification is completed fully, the earliest traces and sources of the initial identification (such as with the moral code of parents) can be decoupled from their source and the object "may somehow be shorn of its quality of otherness and be experienced as part of the essential self" (p. xiii).

This is in contrast to the process of introjection, which "does not aim at likeness, sameness, or merging; it aims to continue a relation with an object, but to displace this relation from the outer world to the inner world" (p. 153). More specifically, Schafer defines an introject as

> an inner presence with which one feels in a continuous or intermittent dynamic relationship. The subject conceives of this presence as a person, a physical or psychological part of a person, or a person-like thing or creature. (p. 72)

An object that has been constituted as an introject "retains its otherness, in which case it will be experienced as a foreign agent, praising, castigating, exhorting, advising . . . to the true inner self" (p. xiiii), but not experienced as "an expression of his subjective self" (p. 72). For Schafer, introjects are also experienced as possessing their own independent motives, and exert "influence" on the subject's motivational system, often compelling or forbidding certain actions or feelings.

For Schafer, objects encountered in external reality are represented psychologically in the mind. The process of introjection begins with the creation of an object-representation. For Schafer, object-representations are "ideas about objects" (p. 28), which are often accompanied by somatic and affective elements which mediate the subject's experience of the object. They range in their degree of verisimilitude and their valence (positive or negative). Multiple representations can be formed and maintained about any given object, with any given level of internal consistency or contradiction (or the lack thereof). As such, for Schafer, when speaking about an "object," we are really discussing the "aggregate" of a given subject's representations of a given object.

In their pure form,[8] objects are experienced, when encountered, as being just "simply there" (p. 123); they are neither inside nor outside, just there. Schafer refers to this as the "indeterminacy of location" (p. 123). Through development and maturation, a child develops the ability to index objects as being either "self" or as being other and external. Relatedly, the child also develops the distinction between an object and its mere representation; the object itself is located externally, while the representation is internal.[9] This differentiation emerges more fully "with the development of reality and logical thinking" (p. 76).

However, some objects are "taken in"; the infant experiences a desire, occasioned by need and crisis, to take in an object and possess it, so that it can maintain an ongoing relationship with it and continue to experience its continuous presence:

> Both the coming into being of an introject and its continued existence represent attempts to modify distressing relations with the object . . . . Introjection continues the subjects attachment to the object, but it does so under a new set of conditions. (pp 73–74)

For Schafer, the paradigmatic illustration of a continued attachment under "new conditions" is that of a child who "takes in" their mother, and feels her continuous *presence* even in her absence; thereby facilitating the child's enduring sense of security and comfort.[10] That is to say, the essential qualities and critical elements of a relationship which generally manifest only in the actual presence of the other object, can, under certain circumstances, emerge in response to the conjured representation of the object, even in its absence. This takes place when the child has the sense that the external object itself, to some degree, has been appropriated by the self.

Indeed, for Schafer, introjection is based on the psychical mechanism of incorporation, which he defines as the sense that one takes in, or intends to take in, "a part or all of another person" (p. 20) into the bodily self. For Schafer, incorporation often has an oral form, and underlies both the processes of introjection as well as identification. In identification, the incorporation aims to acquire some aspect or quality of the other person into the self. Whereas in introjection the aim to transpose the relationship with the other person from a merely external one to an internal one, and thereby to continue the relationship even in the absence of the physical presence of the other. Accordingly, for Schafer, an introject possesses the essential characteristics of the object it is intended to represent.

For Schafer, the process of introjection resembles closely and recapitulates the process described by Freud as "hallucinatory wish fulfillment" (p. 76), in that internal needs lead the child to conjure the object-representation in such a way that the object itself is experienced as present.[11] However, what distinguishes introjection from hallucinatory wish fulfillment is that the process of introjection occurs only *after* the indexing of object location has already taken place, and after the distinction has emerged between object and representation. It therefore involves a change (albeit temporary) in psychological structure, when an object-representation generated internally is no longer indexed as internal, but is experienced again as immediately "present" and real; under these conditions, the boundary between internal and external has been eroded with the collapse of the distinction between object and mere representation. For Schafer, this form of structural change is "regressive" (p. 77), in that it marks a return to an earlier form of psychical representation in which the indexing of location is essentially absent.

Critically, Schafer argues that the distinction between inner and outer is still in and of itself insufficient to explain the essential paradox of introjects.

To put it more directly, how an object can be both internal and external, self and not-self, at the same time? Schafer sets out to resolve this issue, and we outline his approach below.

To resolve this seeming paradox, Schafer begins by suggesting that in parallel to object-representations, there is also a corresponding category of self-representations of the "subjective self," which he defines as what the subject refers to when he says "I, me, myself" (p. 79).

Schafer thus proposes a more nuanced account of the subjective self, and maintains that self-experience can be broken down into three primary modes of experience: the self-as-agent (the I), the self-as-object (the me), and the self-as-place, which does not have a specific pronoun, but is represented in the example of "I feel bad inside" (p. 80). Accordingly, Schafer suggests that the introject can be said to be indexed as an external object that has been internalized into the self-as-place.

Schafer then proceeds to address a second critical issue for the full accounting of introjects; namely, the question of an introject's "influence" (p. 82). For Schafer, the introject's influence is one of the central features of the phenomenon, and one that distinguishes introjects from mere object-representations (which are more ideational in nature). As Schafer describes it, the introject's influence can be experienced with either a negative valence, such as feeling the presence of a sharply critical parent (which generates anxiety or shame) or a positive valence, such as feeling the presence of a comforting object (which generates an experience of warmth and reassurance). Regardless of the valence, the introject is experienced as an autonomous agent, whose presence is either inescapable or near (depending on the valence), and which generates specific, almost visceral, reactions in the subject approximating those which would be experienced in the object's actual presence.

This apparent "influence" presents a similar quandary; if an introject is "essentially a product of the imagination" (p. 83), how can it then alter the subject's moment to moment experience of reality? In order to explain this issue, Schafer proposes an analysis of daydreams, which to his understanding possess key phenomenological similarities to those which he has identified in introjects, and thus provide the resolution to his quandary. Given the centrality of this issue, we will follow this concluding piece of Schafer's account.

Schafer begins by citing Freud's approach to the topic of daydreams, which suggests that the "daydreamer turns away from reality, that he suspends the operation of the reality principle in favor of the pleasure principle" (p. 89). For Schafer, this understanding of daydreams presents two particular conceptual problems. The first problem concerns the nature of the "turning away" from reality and the suspension of reality testing. Schafer argues as follows: it is well-established that the content of daydreams is typically well-grounded in reality testing, often following realistic scenarios and sometimes even beginning to approximate what might be a plan.

Moreover, even though daydreams often feel very real and immediate to the dreamer, they do not involve a genuine detachment from the demands and objects of the external world; as Schafer notes, people often daydream while performing monotonous tasks, and otherwise go about their lives regularly even while daydreaming. Additionally, people often reemerge from daydreams rapidly, even when interrupted. As such, daydreams can hardly be compared to psychotic process; in what sense then is there a suspension of reality testing?

Schafer suggests that in fact, the suspension of reality testing is "neither in the content nor in the context of action" (p. 90). Rather, as Schaffer suggests,

It is when the daydream feels real to him (italics added) that the subject has turned away from reality. (p. 90)

Schafer then proposes to explain the mechanisms through which the day-dreamer experiences the daydream with a sense of immediacy and "reality," despite a general rootedness in objective reality (as reflected in the content and context of typical daydreaming). To do this, he suggests the presence of an additional form of self-representation, one that functions as a "prerequisite to any reality testing" (p. 91). He calls this the "reflective self-representa-tion," (p. 91) in which there emerges in the coding of thoughts an awareness of the self as the "thinker of the thought" (p. 91). Schafer regards reflective this reflective form of self-consciousness as deriving from superego develop-ment, in that it is a form of "self-observation" (p. 107).

For Schafer, it is the internalization of the comments and marked reflec-tions such as "you said this," "you wished that," "you'd better put that other thing out of your mind" made by parental figures "with whom one has identified" (p. 107) that serve as the core of the reflective self-identification. Though its origins are in the superego, it eventually shifts to the ego system once reality testing has become consolidated.

As such, Schafer argues that what happens in a daydream is not a psychotic process (which would be reflected in chaotic and disorganized content), but the unfolding of "regular" nonpsychotic thoughts with a suspension of the reflective self-representation:

The thinker vanishes but the thought remains. Now as an event, a thing, a con-crete external reality, for there is no thinker to know it for what it is. (p. 92)

This suspension of reflective self-representation is, according to Schafer, the essence of primary process thinking in which there is a concreteness and immediacy to thought unmediated by any kind of reflective process or index-ing. Therefore, as Schafer explains, the absence of reflective self-representa-tions in essence renders all thought as primary process.

However, as Schaffer notes, the suspension or absence of reflective self-representations in daydreaming is temporary and easily reversible. Therefore, Schaffer concludes that broadly speaking, the daydreamer maintains his overall commitment to reality testing while experiencing a regression limited in scope.

To illustrate this further, Schaffer takes the example of a paranoid schizo-phrenic "with an organized delusional system" (p. 97), whose reality testing is to a large degree is generally intact in matters not related or incorporated into the specific delusional framework which he has developed. Accordingly, Schafer argues that in such an instance it is more accurate to conceptualize the nature of the psychotic structure as a partial regression in reality testing, brought about by relaxation in a loss of "reflectiveness" (p. 97) surrounding his psychotic ideation or hallucinatory experiences. Schafer suggests that this is also the structure of a daydream, which involves a localized and specific relaxation of reflective self-representation surrounding the images and ide-ation of the daydream. Schafer refers to this phenomenon, present both in some forms of psychosis and in daydreaming, as the "splitting of the ego" (p. 97).

Having laid out this approach to daydreaming, and having explicated his concept of partial regressions, Schafer returns to clarify the nature of introj-ects. He argues that the experience of introjects and their influence is made possible by a similarly regressive shift, a "splitting of the ego," in which the intense desire for the object (at times occasioned by moments of crisis) causes an attenuation of reflective self-representation vis-à-vis the object; such that when its object-representation is conjured, the presence of the representation, or the image of the memory, can be similarly experienced as concrete, real, and immediate. As such, "the introject experience may still be termed a day-dream experience of a specific sort"[12] (p. 112). For Schafer, this explains what allows the self to experience the immediacy of the object while maintaining an ongoing overall rootedness in reality.

Similarly, for Schafer, this process (a conjured object-representation and concomitant suspension of the reflective self-representation) also explains the issue of "influence." Introjects, both gratifying as well as harsh, are essen-tially conjured; they are brought to the foreground of the mind by an intense desire for the object." As such, the introject is cast, so to speak, in a role con-nected to the ongoing drama of the present given moment. Consequently, its apparent influence is in reality nothing more than a product of the self's own needs and wants at the given moment. Accordingly, its demands are coercive only insofar as they are meaningful to the subject, in that they derive from and relate to elements within his own motivational structure. For example, a harsh superego derives its strength from the subject's investment and identification with the essential validity of the demand; the self has a "reason," a motivational purpose, in conjuring the harsh introject in that moment of crisis (perhaps even a masochistic one, see p. 114), and it is this purpose which is in effect exerting pressure on the self, through the conjured character of the introject.[13]

Thus, for Schafer, what seems to emerge is that the term "introjection" has two related connotations. There is the sense of "setting up" introjects, which occurs during childhood, through incorporation; that the child has experienced a certain sense or feeling in relation to a given object (such as warmth or security in the presence of the mother), and has been able to "take it inside" (either the "sense" or the object) and possess it, such that it can be subsequently conjured and reexperienced. These representations have acquired (or retained,) a certain quality which allows for them to be experienced later in life as "immediately present," in moments of crisis or need. And secondly, there are the later regressions in various moments of adult life in which secondary process indexing of location is suspended (through the suspension of the reflective self-representation) and in which the introject is reanimated and reexperienced as present.

Moreover, this process of introjection is essentially one of internalization, since what it accomplishes, as well as what drives it, is a transposition of an external relationship to an internal one, which takes place within the boundaries of the self; the subjective experience of the object as present and the collapse of indexing are the products of a desire to incorporate, to bring in, and to possess an external object or an external relationship and reconstitute it within the self. In sum, when the subject's subsequent responses to the mere representation of the object sufficiently approximate those which arise in response to the actual object,[14] the relationship itself can then be said to have been internalized, such that the relationship with the object itself now continues with its representation. As Schafer explains, these kinds of responses to conjured representations are facilitated by regressions in which indexing of localization has been relaxed. This temporary suspension of indexing is itself a result of the suspension of the reflective self-representation, through a process structurally and functionally similar to wish-fulfilling daydreams.

We have introduced Schafer's rendering of the psychoanalytic approach to the process of internalization with the intention of formulating a developmental framework for an expanded model of Kantian reflective judgment (as proposed in the previous chapter), with the ultimate goal of explicating the phenomenology and symptomatology of compulsive doubting. Taking stock of what we have seen in Schafer, we can suggest the following elements of a developmental framework surrounding judgment.

Our essential thesis is that the development of judgment has roots in the internalization of relationships with significant objects in early childhood. To this end, we draw upon Schafer's presentation of superego development, which allows us to give an account of the acquisition of the substance of categories which guide judgment (as the parameters for subsumption) as well the development of the faculty itself.

To restate Schafer's model briefly, the superego emerges through the process of an internalization of a parental figures; specifically, through the mechanism of identification, the child modifies their subjective self to "become like" the parental figure, resulting in changes to and realignment within the child's motivational system. The outcome of this process is that the motives, aims, and qualities which were previously only that of the parental figure have now been assimilated into the child's subjective self; they now represent a critical aspect of his own motivational system, and are largely de-identified and decoupled from the object-representation itself. However, when identification is incomplete (arising from ambivalence, conflict with other identifications, and the inherent incompleteness of identification), then the demands of the parental figure can be experienced as self-alien.

For Schafer, it seems to emerge that this "self-alien" quality of superego function can take one of two forms, depending on the degree to which the identifications subserving superego development have been "integrated" into the subjective self.[15] When the parental object has otherwise been assimilated to a high degree into the subjective self, the "self-alien" quality of the representation should not be described as an introject. As Schafer suggests, there are times in which an identification may become temporarily self-alien, without losing its status as an identification; for instance, when any given identifications may be in conflict with one another, one of these identifications may be coded as contiguous with the self, while the other may temporarily be experienced as self-alien, and the subjective experience of "me-ness" (p. 18) associated with this identification temporarily recedes. This now self-alien identification may be experienced in any number of ways, including as one which "take[s] on a demand character" (p. 18) toward the self.

However, Schafer suggests that when a given identification is not "well-integrated" (p. 18), the self-alien quality may in fact be properly described as belonging to an introject. Furthermore, some identification may have emerged with objects which have been initially introjected. In these situations, the incompleteness of the identification allows for a re-distillation of an aspect of self back into an external and self-alien motive; and therefore, the identification decomposes back into an introject.

As Schafer suggests, "these ambiguities are often evident during the analysis of superego function" (p. 18), during which "the patient begins to repudiate these strictures and treat them as alien influences" (p. 18). For Schafer, this "repudiation" can either be reflective of a temporary dissociation of "me-ness" from a well-established aspect of self, or a function of the "weakness of true superego formation in many patients" (p. 18) and therefore a more profound decomposition of a tenuous identification back into a self-alien presence, that is, an introject. In this instance, the "self-quality" of the "self-criticism" generated by the superego "may be superficial and misleading" (p. 18, in footnote).

Importantly, it emerges then that Schafer would (under certain circum-stances) describe this self-alien experience of the demanding parental figure (which results from the ambivalence and inherent incompleteness of identi-fication) as a true "introject." Accordingly, we return to consider again some of the basic conditions Schafer outlines (p. 122) for the term "introject." First, the representation of the demanding parental object constitutes the transposi-tion of a relational pattern which existed previously between self and object into one between self and object-representation; the "mere representation" of the object catalyzes the same reactions as does the object itself. Furthermore, under conditions in which identification has receded, the representation of the parental object is not merged with representations of self, either as object or as agent; it remains distinct from and alien to, the subjective self. Nonetheless, since the representation is not hallucinatory, the representation is indexed as "internal" rather external, and is included within the boundaries of the self as location.[16]

Thus, Schafer is articulating the crucial role superego development plays in the internalization of regulatory motives whose initial manifestation lies in the regulatory function of others, outside the self.

However, Schafer also noted Hartmann's earlier position, that the process of internalization is grounded in the "taking in" of schematic information, and formation of a set of rules for what to do and what not to do. It would seem then, that the enlargement of internalization from praxis to motivation should not entail the negation of the informational element, and that both are true; knowledge of the world, as well as regulatory motives, are both assimilated into the self. We attempt to show how both aspects of superego development allow for the transposition of our expanded Kantian framework into that of a psychological (and psychoanalytic) one.

Beginning with the schematic elements of superego development, we sug-gest here, following Parsons (1958), that superego development is not merely the condensation of a system of rewards and punishments restricted to the matrix of the nuclear family, but rather reflects the broader internalization of norms and values of the larger sociocultural environment:

> Most attention has been given to the concept of the superego. . . . there is no
> doubt that it refers to the internalization to become a constitutive part of the

structure of the personality itself, of aspects of the normative culture of the
society in which the individual grows up. (p. 322)

Meaning to say, that for Parsons, the sociological categories of norms
and values are internalized through the psychological process of superego
development.[17]

Returning now to the Kantian framework, we can suggest that the substance of many of the categories which guide subsumption and inform judgment, especially normative and evaluative judgments, is internalized as part
of the process of superego development.

As mentioned, Schafer follows Hartman's expansion of superego internalization, which includes the regulatory function played by the parents in
the guidance of the child's behavior. While Schafer's account emphasizes
the assimilation of "regulatory motives," we can suggest further that what is
internalized in superego development is also a related guiding function that
the parental figures play in the interpretation of reality. That is to say, the
child comes to regard the parent as an object that has a role and a function as
a decider, an arbiter, and a guide. We provide here Shapiro's (2000) description of Werner's (1948) approach to the developmental origins of rigidity,
which he locates within the child's need for external guidance on account of
his incomplete cognitive development, and therefore his reliance on programmatic approaches that show him the "right way" of doing things:

> The child has no clear and objective sense of the relation between action and
> aim, hence an aspect of the situation brings to mind the recollection of the whole
> procedure, the "right way" to proceed. (p. 72)

Shapiro broadens Werner's position and suggests further that this need for
guidance and clarification is what generates the child's acceptance of parental
authority:

> We are accustomed to regarding the young child's unquestioning acceptance
> of adult authority as a natural expression of the child's dependence, and the
> adult's prestige in the child's eyes, but it must reflect the child's lack of a clear
> understanding of the essential elements of a situation. (p. 73)

For Shapiro, then, the child's acceptance of parental authority is not merely
a result of identification; rather, it is the result of an implicit recognition, on
the part of the child, that it needs to rely on the adult's determination of "the
right way to proceed."

It seems indicated to suggest that if, according to Shapiro, the child looks
to the parent as a guide, there is then an experience of the parent as an object

cast in the role of guide, judge, and determiner "of the right way" to go about things. Implicit in this formulation is that in this object-relation, the child expects (and receives) guidance, direction, admonishment, and reassurance; and in return, the parental authority provides a rendering of reality which the child accepts as definitive and relies upon. In essence, then, the child's seeking and receiving the adult's guidance is really a cognitive-affective mode of experience through which the child makes sense of their world. We can say then, that this role of guide and knower of the "right way," can be conceptualized as a regulatory function, subject to internalization through identification. Successful internalization would imply that the child has acquired the tendency of thought, the habit of mind and of experience, to know for themselves and determine for themselves "the right way" to proceed.

In essence, then, we are talking about a capacity to make determinations and judgments, which allows us to link this discussion to Kant's position that judgment is a capacity. We are suggesting then that the Kantian capacity to determine the nature of things, while an innate feature of cognition, is also shaped by the child's experience of parental figures upon whom he must rely to guide his interpretation and navigation of the world. That is to say, that while the ability, in the purely cognitive sense, to subsume particular under universal (even in cases of problematical subsumption) is an innate feature of mind, making determinations and judgments is also something people *do*; it is part of the broader repertoire of how one navigates the world.

In children, both aspects, the cognitive elements as well as the *functional* elements (the concrete performance of the mental processes, which will inform behavior) of judgment and determination are outsourced to adults, upon whom the child relies for guidance. With the child's attainment of cognitive maturity, we can suggest a split between the cognitive and functional aspects of judgment. We can readily imagine a child who is cognitively capable of making a given judgment, for instance, determining whether a given high school is a "good school"; he has a notion of what makes a school good, and he is cognitively capable of determining whether any given school is subsumed under the universal. However, this does not mean that the child necessarily feels that the determination is his to make. He might (and reasonably so) expect his parents to make that determination *for* him, on his behalf. Thus, this conception of the parent, whom he has cast as a knowing and determining figure, may still exist for an older child in much the same way it exists for a younger child. Making this kind of judgment is simply not something he does; it is a function continued to be outsourced to the determining knowing-figure.[18]

In the normal developmental trajectory, the child increasingly performs this function by themselves. Indeed, they will eventually decide where their own children will attend school. Following Schafer, we can say that the child internalizes the determining function performed by the adult; he comes to see it as part of his subjective self-representation, something *which he does*, and he assimilates it into those things that he *actually does* for himself. Through identification with the parental authority, the child assimilates the regulatory function of judging along with the other regulatory functions described by Schafer. He comes to see himself "*as his father*," or "*like his father*," and takes on the roles carried out by the adult.

However, someone who is chronically indecisive may not see this function as something that he does, even as an adult; despite his cognitive capacity to make a given determination, it is not something that he *actually does*, and it is quite likely that he continues to outsource (or attempts to) this function to others, perhaps even to the parental authority of his childhood. He has not, then, assimilated the performance of this function into his way of being. Within the topography of his psychological world (his understanding of himself, and the self in relation to others; as distinct from his cognitive capacities), the function of judgment is one that is to be performed by someone other than himself. He might know, in the abstract, what categories (universals) are germane to a given judgment, but cannot *actually* consistently perform the function of determining.

However, a critical point of clarification still needs to be made here. Though we have posited a process through which judgment is "outsourced," it is not always the case that compulsive doubters seeking reassurance will in fact accept the judgments of those to whom they have turned.[19] To this point, we can suggest that though one may have outsourced the function of judgment (in the sense of making an ultimate determination about something), this does not imply that the evaluative processes (both cognitive and affective), which are at play before ultimate determinations are made, have been inhibited. That is to say, that in the absence of an internal resolution, the OCD doubter experiences ambivalence engendered by the two poles of a given quandary. Accordingly, he may find that while he desires (and expects) the ultimate determination to be made by an external source, this external "judgment" does not result in the resolution of his ambivalence at all. In fact, the judgment's essential externality (when it is made by others on his behalf) may inherently render it unable to resolve inner conflict.

This is, in essence, the model Lazarov et al. (2010) have suggested in the Seeking Proxies model of OCD, where the absence of internal states of subjective certainty and "knowing" lead to a heavy reliance on seemingly objective external markers, as well as reassurance seeking.[20] We are suggesting here that this tendency can be understood within the context of the processes of identification and internalization; that is, an incomplete or insufficient internalization of a parental figure implies a correspondingly incomplete assimilation of the roles and functions performed by that figure into the self. For whatever the reason, the child has not fully come to regard themselves "as" or "like" the parental figure; in the schematic layout of the child's fundamental expectations of the world, the child retains the expectation that this determining function is still to be performed by the adult authority, not by himself.

It is therefore readily understandable why, even as an adult, this expectation remains to a large degree unaltered; it results in a fundamental and pervasive lack of conviction and confidence in one's own faculties of knowing and determining. The adult has retained the same distance (and alienation) from his own perceptions as the child who double-checks with their parent to make sure he is doing something "the right way." He retains the fundamental sense that the quality of "rightness" can only be endowed from outside. Correspondingly, many of his own cognitive processes remain coded with a fundamental tentativeness and a lack of confidence, an uncertainty about whether they are valid and can be relied on.[21] We are suggesting that this tentativeness is not merely metacogntive; it is grounded within the matrix of an object-relation, and derives from conceptions of the self in relation to the parental figure, who (within this object-relation) retains the magical ability to endow things with the quality of "rightness."

Similarly, through this lens we can also address the checking compulsions present in compulsive doubting. Returning again to the doubter who must repeatedly check to see whether he has locked his front door after leaving the house,[22] we can suggest the following approach: what is at stake for the checker is a determination of safety, such that the checker desires to reach a point where he can know definitively that his house is secure and protected. However, this kind of determination is one which he does not feel to be his to make. He remains trapped within the loop of parsing various sensory stimuli; "did the lock make the right noise, indicating a click? It sounded different this time, so perhaps it didn't fully click into place. I might have felt too much resistance when I turned the lock, so perhaps it didn't fully turn?," and so on. What is missing is the movement, described by Beiner, to "to rise above particulars as given in sensory perception" (Beiner, p. 49); to determine definitively that despite missing elements of environmental feedback, the house (and himself as well) is indeed safe. Thinking developmentally, this is precisely part of the determining and reassuring function performed by the parental authority; a child is apt to ask a parent, "do I need to go back and check?" And the parent, in turn, is apt to make their own determination about the safety of the given situation. As such, we can suggest that the predicament of the compulsive checker reflects an incomplete internalization of the parental authority, suggesting that he has not fully assimilated into himself the determining function performed by the parent. It has not been integrated into those regulatory functions which he has mastered and incorporated into his way of being.

Essentially, we are asking how it comes to be that people, within the context of the parent-child relationship described by Shapiro, come to rely on their judgments, to treat their own judgments as sufficient substitutes for those made by the parent, and endowed with the same legitimacy and validity? We are suggesting here that the question of how one learns to rely on their judgments and to trust themselves, is related to the broader question of identification with the parental figure and its subsequent internalization.

At the beginning of the chapter we restated a series of questions pertaining to the nature of self vs. other within the context of judgment. Two of those questions pertained to Kant's notion of the sensus communis. The first of these two concerned the nature of self when making judgments made with the "enlarged mentality" of the sensus communis; how is it that judgments made from the point of view of others (or the universal community) outside the self—feel as if they were made by the self? Following Schafer's topography of the self, we can attempt to clarify this point. If the representation of the sensus communis emerges from a process of internalization (we will return to this point in our discussion of Mead), then we might suggest that the identification with the larger community can lead to a process whereby the communal norms, values, and regulatory motives become integrated and assimilated into his own. As such, while conceptually these have their origin outside of the self, when the subject draws on them to guide his thinking, he is drawing on elements which have become fused into his own character and personality.

Last, Schafer's topography allows us to suggest an approach to the broader phenomenology of compulsions within OCD symptomatology. While we will revisit this point later, we can attempt to explain a perplexing feature of compulsions, which is the quality of a self-alien presence which is directing and requiring the compulsive behavior. What does it mean, and how is it possible, to have a non-self presence within the self and within the mind?

Perhaps, within the phenomenology of OCD compulsions, we are talking about the presence of an introject, and a particularly harsh, demanding, and critical one. Nothing is ever good enough to meet the approval of this introject, which is set up to judge the "rightness" of every action using the most exacting standards of performance. And when inevitably the subject is found wanting, the introject commands for the action to be repeated, again and again, until some unknowable and undefinable point has been reached, and the introject is mysteriously and finally content with the state of things.

This introject would seem to be the same object whose internalization allows for the emergence and crystallization of the superego. It would be, in Schafer's taxonomy, the presence of another within the self-as-place. As such, the compulsions themselves can be other-identified, in the sense that these motives are assigned to the object-representation of a self-alien object, located within self-as-place. Furthermore, by conceptualizing the issuer of the demands as the representation of an essentially foreign object, we can think about an object-relation, and the themes and roles being enacted and repeated (such as harsh judgment, withholding approval) within this relationship.

Having presented Schafer's account of the psychodynamics of internalization, we turn now to look at two theories that highlight aspects of a dialogical consciousness, those of Mead and Vygotsky. A discussion of the dialogical features of consciousness will further illuminate the questions we have posed about the nature of an internalized "other" within the self.

NOTES

1. For Kant, the term refers to the necessary and universal structures of consciousness which make possible the ability to have any meaningful experience at all.

2. In addition to the core of Schafer's theory which we present here, Schafer also attempts to transpose and integrate his model into an economic account in terms of cathexis. Given that his account does not seem dependent on this transposition, our focus will remain on his more structural description.

3. As Schafer explains, these include the development of thought and the emergence of the superego, among other examples.

4. Importantly, Schafer does address the role of ambivalence within the processes of internalization. See his discussion of this issue on p. 17–18, where he describes how ambivalence embedded within identifications can lead to oscillations in the degree to which they are experienced self or self-alien. Elsewhere (see his discussion on pp. 73–74), Schafer suggests that a degree of ambivalence towards the object itself is inherent in both identification and introjection. For Schafer, this is especially the case for introjects, about which he maintains that both their creation and subsequent reemergence "represent attempts to modify distressing relations with the external object" (p. 73).

5. As we have outlined above, identifications can either be mediated by primary process or by secondary process. Accordingly, the "reorganization" of the motivational system can either be experienced consciously (and guided, at least to some extent, with a degree of purposiveness and intentionality), or guided by unconscious (or primary- process) mentation.

That being said, Schafer is clear that at its core, identification "is based on primary-process (ordinarily unconscious) ideation: among other things it includes the idea of fusing or merging with the object, and in this way continuing a relationship with it...it is moved from the external world to the inner world" (p. 161). Nonetheless, while allowing that the wish for merger has "its fantasy aspect," Schafer argues that neither identification nor introjection (which he suggests to be partially rooted in "unconscious primary-process ideation," (p. 78) should be "regarded simply as a fantasy or daydream" (p. 39).

6. See p. 177 where Schafer cites Freud's description of superego development, which dovetails with his own account of progression from identification to relative autonomy.

7. See pages 161–180 for Schafer's full treatment of this issue, and p. 163 for the five lenses he proposes through which to analyze identifications.

8. Schafer concedes that there is an initial state of "unity of self and object" (p. 75), out of which differentiation occurs. Schafer proposes that this stage is followed by one of an "archaic stage of limited differentiation" (p. 75), in which objects exist as distinct but non-localized, and that it is this stage to which regressions often occur. See p. 75 for a fuller outline of Schafer's trajectory of localization.

9. See next note 11 below for a fuller outline of these processes.

10. Schafer here (p. 77) cites Winnicott's description of the infant's ability to maintain its connection to the mother despite her moments of absence or preoccupation.

11. As Schafer explains, this process serves as a platform for scaffolding the child's emerging capacity for reality-testing; since the conjured representation does not result in a reduction of drive-related "need tension" (p. 76), the child begins to distinguish between the object itself and its mere representation. According to Schafer, these representations, located internally, are encoded and organized in secondary process as memory traces of encounters and experiences with external objects. However, under circumstances of intense need for the object, this indexing is removed, and the internal representation can again be experienced as the presence of an external object.

12. Importantly, Schafer seems to categorize the process of introjection as a "wish-fulfilling daydream of another's presence" (p. 111). Moreover, for Schafer, it seems to emerge that the essential mechanism of a daydream itself (what makes it effective at producing gratification and enjoyment) is that the self "chooses," in a way, to relax and suspend the self-representation, with the aim of generating an experience which is "real and gratifying" (p. 111).

13. Importantly, though it is outside the scope of our discussion, see Schafer's discussion (p. 129–130) of the possible connection between introjects and the process of projection.

14. These include the child's sense of security and comfort arising in response to the conjured representation of the mother in a manner which to some degree approximates the sense which emerges in response to the actual mother. It is in this way that the child has "taken in" and incorporated the qualities of the mother (or the relationship to her) which he so desperately needs.

15. See pages 17–18 for Schafer's presentation of this issue. Schafer's delineation of the specific "ambiguities" described on page 17, his elaboration that they are dependent on the degree of integration of a given identification, and the link to specific permutations of self-alien qualities of superego functioning are somewhat terse, especially the latter point. What appears below is an attempt at a more systematic reading of his account and its implications.

16. This account is not at odds with Schafer's position that there is no need to maintain a "temporal precedence" of mediating introjects during the process of identification (p. 19), since our discussion of the superego involves a specific regressive shift in structure from identification to introject, in which something previously experienced as part of the self becomes experienced as something self-alien.

17. Indeed, as Parsons describes, the internalization of norms and values happens through the internalization and resolution of relationships within the nuclear family.

18. This of course does not obviate a give and take between the child and parents surrounding the choice; in this particular example, we are emphasizing the child's awareness of the comparatively greater responsibility borne by the parents regarding his decision, such that he understands that their input is also critical for his own thinking and for his own confidence, and that they too must "sign off" on his choice.

19. In fact, it is well known that reassurance seeking can often be an almost unending process. See for instance Huppert et al. (2007).

20. See note 3 in the Introduction.

21. We will revisit these points about tentativeness and the sense of the fundamental legitimacy of one's own judgments and perceptions in our discussion of Winnicott, below.

22. This would be true for symmetry checking as well, since these are also judgments and determinations.

Chapter 3

The Self as the Other

Mead's Account of Internalization and the Emergence of the Self

In the previous chapter, we raised two questions about the nature of the sensus communis: 1) how does one develop the "enlarged mentality" of the sensus communis, and 2) what allows for the subject to experience, as his own, judgments which are rooted in the expected and anticipated responses of external figures and grounded in external norms? In response, we proposed that the process of internalization is critical to explaining how the sensus communis becomes developmentally constituted in the mind. In this chapter, we will use Mead's model of the self to address this question, and suggest a further developmental grounding for this Kantian feature of mind. In particular, we will draw from Mead's notion of the "generalized other," which will be central to our discussion. In order to do so, we must first lay out and describe the critical building blocks of Mead's approach, which will allow us properly present his full theory.

We now turn then to a discussion of Mead's model of the self. This will involve us in three areas of Mead's work. The first issue concerns the central distinctions between human and animal social organization. The second is Mead's theory of language and communication. And lastly, the third issue, and the one most critical for our discussion, is Mead's theory of the social and developmental origins of the self. For Mead, the proper articulation and resolution of all these issues is rooted in an analysis of certain particular features of human consciousness and the nature of thought. Given that Mead's treatment of these issues take place in a range of different papers, we present here an integrated overview and outline of these discussions as they appear in three of Mead's works[1]: The Problem of Society, (1936), The Process of Mind in Nature, (1938), and the collection of edited papers titled Mind, Self, and Society (1934).

In his paper The Problem of Society, Mead intends to explicate the under-lying mechanisms in human societies that facilitate social control. We begin with this discussion because it allows us to introduce Mead's notion of "atti-tudes" and his particular agenda of locating human consciousness and self-consciousness within the sphere of human social behavior.

Mead begins by noting that human social organization is fundamentally different than that of the animal world; human societies are distinct even from animal systems of high complexity and coordination, such as those found in ants and bees. This is so because for the participants in human society there is an attitudinal and self-conscious identification with the norms and values of the larger community that informs the actions of the individual. This is in contrast with the "the social control which results from blind habit" (p. 35) which governs the unthinking social behaviors of the animal world, even in systems with a high degree of complexity.

Essentially, for Mead, what differentiates human societies from animal societies in terms of their social coordination is not necessarily their degree of complexity but rather the quality of their coordination. Whereas animals act mechanically and instinctively and reflexively respond to environmental stimuli, human beings *consciously choose* to fulfill the roles and perform actions that are expected of them. This quality of identification is what accounts for the unique aspect of human social control, which is marked by the tendency of one to "admonish himself as others would" (p. 35). Identification ultimately produces a full involvement of the individual within the social order, both to admonish himself, as well as "recognize what are his duties as well as what are his rights" (p. 35), and therefore becomes a catalyst for purposive and self-conscious behavior.

For Mead, this capacity for social organization is made possible through the use of language. The full impact of this will be explained more fully below later in the summary of Mead's theory of language, but it suffices for now to say that for humans, the link between stimulus and response is mediated by consciousness (mind). Mead argues that this must be so because of the inherent ambiguity of the total field of the environment, which often presents ambiguous stimuli which require interpretation. Additionally, human beings must also sift through a range of possible behavioral responses to any given stimulus. Whereas animals often respond to stimuli reflexively (as their responses are often directly stimulated by odor and touch; and are therefore more clearly neurobiological and conditioned), the responses of human beings are more complex. They involve thought, reflection, inhibi-tion, and planning, and cannot be reduced to simple conditioning processes. Additionally, as we will see, Mead highlights the necessity and capacity for behavioral inhibition, which he takes as further evidence for the view that consciousness itself is needed for a full account of behavior.

For Mead, this conscious control of behavior is instantiated in the mind through processes of reasoning; in terms of stimuli, the mind works to interpret the meaning of stimuli, as well as parse out the elements of the presentation and environment which are critical and salient for a response; the signal from the noise, so to speak. At the other end, it is the process of reasoning through the range of outcomes and the range of possible behaviors in response to the stimulus which allows for a determination of the best course of action in a given situation. For Mead, reasoning is essentially a thought process, expressed in language; and language, in turn, implies communication. Thus, for Mead, thought is essentially an internal conversation, a reflexive form of communication in oneself and with oneself.

However, Mead argues further that communication through language implies an additional aspect of human thought: that the use of language for social communication rests on the capacity for "taking the attitude" (p. 38) and perspective of the other or the community. He proceeds to analyze an example (which recurs in his writing, and that we will revisit as well) of someone who observes a fire, and shouts out "fire!" Mead analyzes it as follows: When one has the thought "fire," the thought is language-based: he is thinking about a word. Meaning to say, he is interpreting visual and environmental stimuli within the framework of the social world, in which the word signifies something; here, it signifies that this stimulus is dangerous, and that the indicated response to this stimulus is to run away.[2] Accordingly, when he shouts "fire," the substance and intention of his communication is to warn everyone else and encourage *them* to run away. Mead argues that this process necessarily makes recourse to an attitudinal element; he is adopting the community's attitude toward the stimulus, that it is indeed dangerous, and that the correct response is in fact to run away. He is also taking the position, psychologically, of the larger community to whom he is talking. He sees things from their perspective. He is able to put himself in their place, such that he understands that they will be in danger, and that they need to run away. As such, when he communicates with them, he is talking not merely from his own internal vantage point, but from having entered theirs: "he is taking the attitude of the other people whom he is directing" (p. 38).

For Mead, there are essentially four points here: 1) that social coordination rests on individuals adopting shared values and attitudes; 2) that any given individual must also be able to enter into the perspective of any other in order to guide and coordinate the behavior of the larger group; 3) that in the process of an individual "figuring out what to do" in any given situation (including the recognition that he must guide others), there is an interpretative process (which Mead identifies as "thought," as we will discuss shortly) through which the individual parses out the meaning of a given environmental stimulus in order to formulate his actions; 4) that this interpretative process of necessity requires "taking the attitude of the other" toward the stimulus, since the functional meaning of the stimulus is culturally known and determined (in the broadest sense of culture, referring to the body of accumulated knowledge about the world stored and transmitted by a group of people).[3]

Having laid this out that thinking involves taking the attitude and the perspective of the other, Mead returns to a discussion of the nature of human thought and restates his central thesis that thought is a reflexive and dialogical process taking place within the self:

> Thinking is a process of conversation with one's self when the individual takes the attitude of the other. (p. 38)

Mead continues further, and describes the nature of thought as "the importation of outer conversation ... into the self" (p. 42). This raises a question, however; if thought is dialogical and reflexive within the self, what actually is the nature of this conversation? And in what way is it modeled after conversation between others? Mead describes this conversation in terms of the thoughts and inner speech which unfold as one is trying to problem-solve. He proposes the following example of what a reflexive "back and forth" might look like in the mind, and what function it serves in behavior: suppose that in the process of directing others, someone raises an objection to the direction; the director would then engage with the objector, either agreeing with him, disagreeing with him, or overruling him. Mead argues that this happens all the time internally; a person has a thought about something, and then another thought comes into his mind contradicting, objecting to, or questioning that original thought; and then another thought arises in response to that thought, and so on. For Mead, that process is essentially a conversation in one's mind, where the person is shifting perspectives between "himself" and a mentalized other, who is objecting: this shifting of perspectives is the "process which we call thought" (p. 38).

As we will describe more fully later in the summary, when the self takes the position of the objector, it has done so by adopting the attitude of the community; one judges his own thoughts, impulses, and environmental responses through the lens of the attitudes of the community (what Mead later refers to as the "generalized other"). Ultimately, Mead proposes further refinements and explications of the internal dialogue, culminating in his famous distinction between the "me" and the "I." These will be revisited in due course, and are the central point of connection to our discussion about Kant's sensus communis. As such, we continue to lay out the points of Mead's thinking in order to appropriately render the link between his line of reasoning and Kant's discussion of the sensus communis.

Before continuing to present Mead's formal theory of language, it is critical to first provide a more detailed analysis of the distinct features of Mead's view of self-consciousness upon which the theory rests. To do so, we continue our overview with Mead's paper Mind in Nature, in which he more formally defines the parameters and features of human self-consciousness, and also expands his conceptualization of reason within the framework of behavioral analysis and S-R (stimulus-response) terminology.

In this paper, Mead argues that an analysis of human behavior within the total environment of objects and stimuli necessitates the existence of a "self," which transcends the contingencies of mechanical and rote responses to stimuli. To make this argument, Mead (p. 98) shows how the human being not only reacts to his environment, but also actively interprets it, apprehends it, and ultimately reshapes it. In this sense, Mead's position anticipates the central arguments of the cognitive revolution and its rejection of Watson's behaviorism (see Reisberg, 2007, for a succinct description of the features of the cognitive revolution).

There are two points made in this paper which are critical for our account. The first is Mead's formulation of self-conscious behavior, and the second is his account of how the human mind is actively involved in the constitution and apprehension of the environmental field.

Mead begins by proposing a definition of self-consciousness:

the individual in acting with reference to the environment should, as part of that action, be acting with reference to himself, so that his action would include himself as an object. (p. 95)

The effect, or advantage of this "action with reference to himself" is a particular kind of environmental learning, one in which, through the process of "reflection" (p. 96), the individual is able to transcend the constraints of mechanical and rote learning which constitute the parameters of trial and error methods.

At the beginning of trial and error tasks, there is often no clear understanding of the internal logic and mechanics of a task. Mead provides the following conceptual formulation, in terms of stimulus and response, to the initial state of confusion: he cannot represent himself in his mind and consciousness "as responding to a specific stimulus in a definite fashion" (p. 96), and as such, is often fumbling about until he begins to have a clearer sense as to how to proceed.

Mead contrasts the difficulties inherent in trial and error learning with the type of learning in which an individual uses their past experiences to make sense of a current task. Mead again provides a behavioral framework through which to articulate this kind of learning. He suggests that when one is able to draw from previous experience, it means that for him "stimulus and response define each other clearly" (p. 97). Mead provides the example of an individual who is walking along a path and comes across a chasm.[4] In this example, the individual's initial response is to try and jump over it; however, he realizes from past experience that it is too wide, and concludes that he cannot make it across by jumping (this example, too, is recurring and we will revisit later in our discussion. In Mead's essay Mind, Self, and Society, he describes the example more fully (p. 184), and our presentation here follows his more expansive description). In this task of crossing the chasm, the individual has a clear sense of the stimulus task, which is to cross the chasm, and its relation to a definite response (jumping); he can formulate to himself and simulate the outcome of response x to stimulus y.

Mead argues that this realization is only possible because of a particular form of self-consciousness that allows him to recall *himself* and conceive of *himself* as an object, set aside from the particulars of his current experience. Moreover, it is only through this form of reflexive self-representation (conceiving of the self as an object, which is the basis for self-consciousness) that a self can maintain a coherent sense of its own history. In other words, it is self-consciousness which allows for the essential experience of stable and continuous selfhood which transcends time and place, and thus serves as the basis through which one can meaningfully access their own memories.

We continue further with Mead's example of the man attempting to cross a chasm. Once the individual realizes that the jumping response is unsuitable to the task-stimulus (of proceeding with the journey), what is likely to happen next? The individual is likely to proceed in any number of different directions; he might notice, looking into the distance, that the width of the chasm is narrower in certain places, and he might walk over to evaluate whether he is able to cross there. Or, he might notice that there are a number of felled trees in the proximity, and he might think to try and use them to bridge the chasm.

Essentially, for Mead, there are four critical stages that take place in this sequence. The first is that the individual can recognize consciously that there is a need to formulate a new plan of action. Implicit in this is that the human being has the kind of cognitive flexibility to recognize and accept that his course of action has not been successful. Whereas a lower order animal would simply disengage from a task after the experience of failure,[5] a human is able to acknowledge that his response is ineffective, reflect on the situation, and reorganize it in his mind. This leads to the second stage in the sequence. One can reflect on why his actions have not been successful; he can isolate elements of his environment, endowing them with new salience, and use them to plan a different course of action then the one he had been pursuing until now.

Mead refers to the processes in this stage as "reflection" and "adjustment," whereby the individual, through the process of reasoning, can come to isolate the particular elements of the stimulus or task that are impeding his progress; he can thereby refine his understanding of the parameters of task-stimulus, as well as his approach to solving the problem itself.

Crucially, Mead also points out another element which is critical for the processes of reflection and adjustment, and that is the mechanism of behavioral inhibition. Returning again to our example, Mead argues that while the individual's initial reaction might be to try and jump over the chasm, he is able to inhibit the response and override his impulse, through the exercise of his self-conscious awareness of its futility or detrimental consequences.

This leads us to the third stage in the behavioral analysis, which is that the individual is able to scan their environment and notice new elements of the environment, which in turn stimulate the propagation of new responses and plans of action. Mead refers to this process as "indicating to himself the stimulus" (see for instance p. 172), such that the individual is able to reinterpret various environmental features into new task-related stimuli which call forth reconfigured responses. Thus, the meaning of a fallen tree can be reappraised, and it moves from being an obstacle in his path to a means to bridge the chasm. Having attained this new meaning and salience, the tree now becomes the task-stimulus for a new set of behavioral responses; lifting the tree, repositioning it, determining its strength, and so on.

The fourth point is that the mind can think through and reason through potential responses; one can represent various potentialities and outcomes simultaneously, and play out multiple plans of actions. This allows him to choose which one is best. Mead argues that this ability is predicated on self-consciousness, in which one conjures themselves, as an object, in their simulation of a response. That is to say, the ability to simulate these responses is contingent on the ability to conceive of the self as an object, such that one can conjure and visualize themselves as the actor within each of the various behavioral responses.

Relatedly, Mead argues that our "ideas" about the "meanings of things" (p. 99) (and therefore the very basis of language of itself) are predicated upon this ability to conceive of the self as an object and as the actor within a set of environmental responses. He provides the example of a chair: we identify the object of the chair with the word "chair," which has a universal meaning, namely, something that you can sit on. For Mead, the ability to apprehend a "chair" in the environment involves then the projected simulation of imagining oneself sitting in it. That is to say, one thinks of a given object as a chair if he can imagine himself sitting in it. As he explains, a word may often refer to a specific response (or set of responses) to a specific environmental stimulus. Accordingly, an accurate apprehension of the stimulus will then involve the conjuring of the corresponding response. This "conjuring," in turn, involves the conception of the self as an object, acting within the environmental field.

At this point, we can now turn our attention to Mead's formal theory of language, drawn from his papers in Mind, Self, and Society. He begins his account by justifying the place for an analysis of language within social psychology. To do this, he introduces his own framework of behavioral analysis which we will define shortly. Mead contends that "no very sharp line can be drawn between social psychology and individual psychology" (p. 115). Rather, the focus of social psychology should be on studying the ways in which societies and social groups shape the attitudes and behaviors of individuals. Moreover, for Mead, it is the social dimension which shapes the contours of individual experience, and therefore social groups cannot be thought of as a mere composite of the individual psychologies of their members.

As we have mentioned, Mead, unlike Watson, takes the position (p. 119), that consciousness is meaningful, and that it plays a central role in behavior. As such, Mead argues that any analysis of behavior cannot rely on splitting what is observable from what is psychological:

Social psychology is behavioristic in the sense of starting off with an observable activity. . . . but it is not behavioristic in the sense of ignoring the inner experience of the individual—the inner phase of that process or activity . . . the act then . . . has both an inner and outer phase, an internal and external aspect. (p. 122)

Thus for Mead, the psychological organization of the act, which catalyzes the coordination and initiation of observable behavior, should be understood as an "inner phase" of the act itself. Mead provides an example of someone preparing to mount a horse, in which the actual initiation of the motor program, such as the tensing of muscles and the positioning of the body, precludes a simple dichotomy between planning and behavior.

Accordingly then, Mead (p. 116) proposes the viewpoint of "social behaviorism," a broad behaviorism defined as "an approach to the study of experience of an individual from the point of view of his conduct, particularly, but not exclusively the conduct as it is observable by others" (p. 116).

Having broadened the parameters of phenomena which constitute "behavior," and having widened the scope of his analysis of behavior within the social context, Mead now lays out his theory of language. As we will shortly see, Mead's analysis of language is grounded within a larger analysis of behavior and consciousness. The rudimentary outline of his theory is that gestures, when communicated from one person, bring about the modification and adjustment of another's behavior. Some gestures are "significant" (p. 168), in that they make use of language. The use of language in turn implies self-consciousness, in that "one must know what he is saying" (p. 205). The presence of this self-consciousness then implies intentionality, in that one person intends to bring about the adjustment of the other's behavior. In Mead's analysis, this intention also implies the ability to take the perspective of the other into account. Ultimately, for Mead, the use of language becomes internalized as thought, while retaining its communicative properties. We present a more thorough treatment of these steps below:

1) For Mead, the basic unit of language is the "gesture." The gesture itself is the means of communicating an attitude, which we have defined as the dispositional readiness to perform a given behavior. Thus, Mead argues that offering a chair to someone to sit down in is a gesture, in that its purpose is communicative; one communicates an attitude of readiness to help and to attend to the other's needs, thereby signaling respect and esteem. As Mead describes, an attitude of politeness is implicit, and can be almost instinctive. As such, the expression of this attitude through gestures (like offering a chair) means that communication itself can be not only non-verbal, but also preverbal.

2) The second aspect of gestures is that in addition to the communication of attitudes, their intention is to evoke an adjustment, or modification, of the behavior of the other person. That is, the essence of communication is to effect some change in another person (see pp. 127–128, in footnote).

Importantly, for Mead, both communication itself as well as coordinated social behavior are expressed within the framework of S-R terminology, such that the gesture is intended to serve as a stimulus to effect a response in another person. This is reflective of Mead's "social behaviorism," which includes social interaction within the framework of behavioral analysis. This point will also be important for the process of the internalization of language.

3) The *meaning* of a gesture can only be understood by reference to the intended modification or adjustment it will effect. As such, the meaning of a gesture is not a "psychical addition" (p. 163), but rather has an objective definition, located within the behavioral field of stimuli and response coordinated between organisms. As Mead explains, "The adjustive response of the other organism is the meaning of the gesture" (p. 168).

4) While some gestures are preverbal and derive from implicit attitudes, much of human communication is self-conscious; meaning to say, that one "is aware of what he is saying" (p. 205). Mead refers to such gestures as "significant gestures" (see for instance p. 168).

For Mead, language is a significant gesture, because the meaning of the gesture is shared between the two parties involved in the communication, such that through the expression of the gesture each party represents the same meaning in their respective minds.

5) Communication through language implies then that there is an intention, through the expression of gesture X, to evoke response Y in another person.
6) Mead now suggests a series of elements which make possible the use of language in order for one to bring about an adjustment on the part of the other. These relate to Mead's assertion that through the use of language, one necessarily "tak[es] the attitude of the other" (p. 159).

Mead is essentially making the following argument:

I.   a gesture is a means to alter another's behavior.
II. language, as a significant gesture, implies self-consciousness and intentionality.
III. this intentionality (to use word x to elicit behavior y) implies an internal simulation of the attempted communication; one represents, in the mind, the communication of the word-stimulus, as well as the anticipated response.
IV. this simulation, therefore, requires an understanding of the effect the word-stimulus is expected to have on the target of the communication; whether it will effect in the other the requisite attitude (defined as the dispositional readiness to engage in any given behavior) toward the desired behavior.
V.   This ability to anticipate and simulate the attitude of the other in response to the word-stimulus is based on one's own awareness of the meaning of the gesture. That is to say, one knows the meaning of the given word-stimulus based on his own reactions to the word; he determines the expected outcome of the gesture based on how he would react if he himself was the other. As such, he is anticipating his own expected attitude toward the word-stimulus.[6]

There is here another related point, which will be important for Mead's discussion of the internalization of language as thought. Mead describes a person who apprehends a dangerous stimulus and seeks to warn others:

> If one calls out quickly to a person in danger, then he himself is in the attitude
> of jumping away, though the act is not performed. (p. 174)

What Mead seems to be saying here goes a step further than merely talking about anticipation and simulation; he seems to be saying that the individual is actually themselves aroused by the apprehension of the danger stimulus. In the process of interpreting the stimulus, he directly represents its meaning to himself; he knows that one must run from fire, so seeing a fire evokes the attitude of running. Subsequently, he may determine that he himself is safe, and does not need to run. Nonetheless, through his awareness that *someone else* is likely still in danger, his attention remains on the need for running in response to the fire-stimulus. In this sense, he is not merely simulating the attitude, but possesses the attitude himself.

Moreover, Mead also suggests instances in which the communicated gesture is intended to elicit a given outcome *x*, and the gesturer includes himself within the set of people intended to have the requisite attitude for behavior *y* (which will produce the target outcome). For instance, if one notices an elderly person walk into a room and announces, "let's get him a chair to sit down," he shares the same attitude of *getting the chair* which he hopes to elicit in the others who are present; he might even get the chair himself if no one else does.

Similarly, it bears repeating again here the point which we noted earlier, that for Mead, the very act of interpreting the stimulus means thinking about it (and therefore using language-based thought) through the universal perspective, that is, the meaning attached to it by the community.

To this point of our discussion, we have laid out a series of points in Mead's thinking. We have outlined his exposition of rational self-consciousness and his theory of language. We can now proceed to lay out how for Mead language becomes internalized, and then present Mead's theory of the self.

We begin by returning to Mead's notion of the processes of "reflection" (Mead also uses the broader term "reflective intelligence") and "recognition," whereby an individual self-consciously directs his attention to the analysis of various environmental stimuli, with the aim of formulating novel responses to navigate an impasse. For Mead, the newly acquired salience of a given stimulus within the context of a novel response derives from a reflexive "calling out" or "pointing out" of the stimulus and its potentialities to one's self. Mead suggests that this process of "pointing out" to oneself is the essence of thought:

"thinking is pointing out—to think about a thing is to point it out before acting" (p. 171, in footnote). That is to say, the process of articulating something to oneself, making explicit to oneself what has until now been implicit and unarticulated, is in essence a reflexive and self-directed process of guiding one's attention and focus toward the various elements of an object which possess a certain salience for a given task. In doing so, the individual allows these stimuli to guide the unfolding of his thoughts as well as his behaviors.

Accordingly, Mead argues that thought is essentially a reflexive process, in which the self is both subject and object; it both initiates communication, as well as receives it. The self communicates reflexively, as if it were talking to another; the self is thereby cast in the role of the other in thought. It calls and directs its own attention to salient stimuli, both internal and external.

Mead further broadens his account of thought, integrating gesture, meaning, and language. He considers a case in which one begins to say something critical or demeaning about another person, but then "realizes it is cruel" (p. 205), and cuts himself short, declining to finish his comment. For Mead, this process illustrates a process of reflexive adjustment, where one responds to their own gestures. Moreover, it also illustrates the ways in which this reflexive "conversation of gestures" (p. 205) can unfold internally, within the self, as thought. That is, the effect of words which are thought is the same as words which are spoken; they both prompt reactions (adjustments and modifications). In thought, one reacts to oneself, by thinking another thought in response to the previous thought, and so on. It is in this way that thought is an internal "conversation of gestures" (p. 205).

Having laid out Mead's theory of the mind, we can now turn to his account of the self. Mead begins by noting that "we can distinguish very definitely between the self and the body" (p. 200); for instance, losing parts of the body may not damage the integrity of the self. Moreover, the distinction between self and body is also represented in the capacity to become absorbed in fantasy and reverie, to the point that one can feel themselves to be in an entirely different place than they are in, with an entirely different set of sensations than those actually within the field of their environment.

Having made a case for the existence of the self, as distinct from the body, Mead now poses the following question: *self-consciousness* means taking the self as an object, in the sense that one is observing themselves; but in order to be *self-conscious*, one must be inhabiting the self, so to speak. This creates a seeming problem, because it leads to the collapse of object into subject; how can one experience the immediacy of selfhood as a subject, while simultaneously experiencing the self as a distant object which he is observing?

The solution Mead suggests is that these modes of self-experience are sequential; there is a continuous oscillation between self as subject and self as object. For Mead, this oscillation is expressed in the process of language-based thought; it is through the reflective and reflexive process of responding to one's thoughts that one transitions from subject to object. One regards their initial thought, which was the product of a subjective self-experience, marked by a sense of "being inside" his own experience, and reacts to it; one evaluates the thought from a position of objectivity, judging it from the point of the view of the universal community. It is through this process that one takes an objective position vis-à-vis his own subjectivity.

To these different oscillating modes of experience, Mead suggests drawing a distinction between "I" and "me." The essential distinction is that the "I" corresponds to the subjective experience of the self, whereas the "me" refers to the self when experienced as an object.

While the parameters of the "me" are more readily accessible, Mead provides the following illustration, clarifying the nature of subjective self-experience and the ensuing transition to objectivity:

> I talk to myself, and I remember what I said and perhaps the emotional content that went with it. The "I" of this moment is present in the "me" of the next moment. . . . I become a "me" insofar as I remember what I said . . . . It is what you were a second ago that is the "I" of the "me." (p. 229)

That is to say, the "I" is the spontaneous, emergent experience of self. It is the actual manifestation of the self in the external world; the mode of active participation, through behavior, in the total environment. Though for Mead, human consciousness is distinguished by its faculties of reason and its capacity for planning, he nonetheless maintains that there is a gap between the planning and reasoning mode of the self, and the active mode of the self, which allows for spontaneity:

> it is because of the "I" that we say we are never fully aware of what we are, that we surprise ourselves by our own action. it is as we act that we are aware of ourselves. (p. 229)

> we are aware of ourselves, and of what the situation is, but exactly how we will act never gets into experience until after the action takes place. (p. 232)

What Mead seems to be saying is that with the transition from the observing mode of self to the active mode of self, there is a diminishment of self-consciousness and self-awareness; the active mode of self-experience implies a move away from observation and evaluation, during which one has less access to the observing perspective through which one normally represents his reasons for doing things. While of course there are reasons that explain his action, they are not fully knowable to him before he acts, and can only be understood in retrospect. The representation of these reasons is not part of the "experience" of the action itself, since the experience of acting is fundamentally different from that of apperception. For Mead, the awareness of the action itself is essentially represented only in memory (importantly, this oscillation between phases does not imply any diminishment of one's volition and will; see note 7 for a fuller explanation of this point).[7]

Mead also defines the "I" in reaction to the "me," by integrating the transitions between these modes of self into his framework of gesture, attitude, and response. For Mead, the "me," as the objective, observing, and planning phase of the self, derives its objectivity from taking on the attitudes of the broader community:

> the "me" is the organized set of attitudes of others which one himself assumes. The attitudes of others constitute the organized "me." (p. 230)

One then evaluates their own impulses and actions from the objective and universal standpoint of this "set of attitudes," which Mead refers to later as the "generalized other" (which will be described more fully below).

The "I" itself emerges in reaction and response to what the self, as the "me," renders as the objective, external, world:

> He had in him all the attitudes of others, calling for a certain response; that was the "me" of the situation, and his response is the "I." (p. 231)

> the me represents a definite organization of the community there in our own attitudes and calling for a response. (p. 233)

Mead further explains how the "I" emerges in reaction to the "me." He suggests that in any given situation, one represents in consciousness an organized group of potential responses. These then in a sense become reflexive stimuli, calling forth some action from the "I"; it is the "me" then which mediates (and interprets) the environmental stimuli, which call out the responses of the "I." Again, for Mead, what that action ultimately will be is not knowable by the self, until it actually occurs, when it is apprehended by the "me."

Mead illustrates this last point by reference to a baseball player, who is in the process of reacting to a ball hit toward him. He has some sense of what he wants to do, or should do, given his positional responsibilities. He intends to catch it, or throw it to another fielder, etc. In a sense, these anticipatory expectations form the player's "me." However, the player's actual response is unknown, even to himself. He may or may not be able to make the play; it may be "a brilliant play or an error" (p. 230). Thus, the player's actual reaction to the ball is a spontaneous event, which could not have been clearly predicted. In this sense, the "I" emerges in action (or reaction) as a spontaneous expression of the individual self. There are of course reasons why the player either makes a brilliant play or an error; perhaps the ball slips out of his hands, the sun blinds his eyes, and so on. But these reasons are only represented in consciousness (and therefore only accessed) after the action itself, as it becomes represented as a memory image.

Importantly, for Mead, individuality is nonetheless still possible despite the assumption of the attitudes of the other: This is so because every individual self occupies a specific position within any given social organiza-tion. Accordingly, though each person internally represents the "organized set of attitudes" (p. 230) of the broader community, they do so from their own "particular and unique place or standpoint" (p. 230). Though all members of a social organization may share the same internalized attitudes and shared sense of the parameters for behavior and action, each individual's specific behavioral response to any given situation will emerge from the particu-larities of their distinct circumstances, roles, and locations within the broader community.

The total picture, then, for Mead is that "me" and "I" are both aspects of the self and modes of experience. They galvanize and catalyze each other in an ongoing process which constitutes the nature of mind and self. For Mead, "the self is essentially a social process" (p. 233) which unfolds through the interaction between these different aspects of the self.

Importantly, for our discussion, Mead identifies the "me" with the Freudian superego, which he refers to as "a censor"[8]: Accordingly, impulsivity can be expressed as the spontaneous "I" expressing itself against the "me," in the sense that his actions and behaviors do not sufficiently take into account the attitude of others in the group, as constituted in the "me." Conversely, social control is achieved through the moderating influence of the "me" against the impulses of the "I."

Mead's position is that the self, with its two phases and modes of expe-rience, is a product of development; specifically, the particular features of reflexivity constituted in these two phases, and instantiated in the pat-terns and flow of thought itself, emerge from the individual's process of socialization. We present here an overview of Mead's account of the self's development.

For Mead, the central element of this process is the capacity for role-play. Accordingly, Mead presents an analysis of role-playing in children, from within the framework of reflexive gesturing (the calling out in oneself) and taking the attitude of the other which are at the core of his theory. Mead notes that for children, role-playing need not take place with others; it can be observed as a process taking place within the child himself. For instance, "the invisible, imaginary, companions" (p. 214) that accompany many children indicate a psychological organization in which the responses they call out in others are also "called out in themselves" (p. 214). Additionally, at times, the child might play both roles by himself, such as playing cashier in a store, in which he acts first as customer presenting money, and then the cashier taking it. In this way, he acts as the other in response to his own self, and takes in the attitudes and responses of the given role, organizing them into "a certain whole" (p. 215). Importantly, for Mead, this kind of role-playing often has a didactic function and facilitates learning about the designated roles within a given social organization, such as mother, fireman, policeman, and so on.

Mead observes that following this more basic form of role-play, more complex role-playing emerges. He argues that these more complex forms of role-play are implicit in children's ability to coordinate with each other in the play of more complex games, like baseball, where "the child taking one role must be ready to take the role of everyone else" (p. 215). He explains that in a baseball game, each player on the field must know, and at times represent, the roles and responses of every other player on the field. For instance, in order to plan his own response, he must anticipate who will catch the ball and what that player will do with it, who will throw the ball and to whom he will throw it, and so on. In this sense, any given player at any given moment takes the attitude of a range of the other players on the field.

At this point then, we have seen how a child develops the ability to represent and maintain in consciousness the roles (as an organized system of attitudes and responses) and perspectives of others. However, Mead argues that still, the child is not yet a "fully developed self," (p. 216) even after learning how to play baseball: "He does not organize his life as we would like to have him do, namely, as a whole." (p. 216). Meaning to say, he takes on roles temporarily, for the purposes of the game. However, he does not reliably stay "in-character" and conduct himself more generally according to systematized roles (which is for Mead the essence of adult life). Nonetheless, for Mead, participating in this kind of game represents a pivotal point in the child's ability to take on the roles and attitudes of others, first in play and then eventually within a stable and systematized social role later in development.

Eventually in the child's development, all the relevant social roles are mastered, integrated, and organized into a coherent and stable pattern of perspectives, roles, and values; in other words, the child, as he transitions into the adult world, develops a coherent character. There is a dependability, consistency, and stability in the adherence to roles and maintenance of attitudes across temporal and situational permutations.

For Mead, the integration of the various roles results in the formation of a "generalized other":

> The organized community or social group which gives to the individual his unity of self can be called "the generalized other." The attitude of the generalized other is the attitude of the whole community. (p. 218)

As Mead makes clear (and as we alluded to earlier), it is the "generalized other" through which the mind attains its capacity for objectivity, and with whom the reflexive dialogue of thought takes place:

We have said that the internal conversation of the individual with himself in terms of words or significant gestures—the conversation which constitutes the process or activity of thinking—is carried on by the individual from the standpoint of the "generalized other." (p. 220, in footnote)

For Mead, as thought becomes more abstract, the "generalized other" also takes on an increasingly abstract quality, and becomes largely independent from "any connection with particular individuals" (p. 220, in footnote). And furthermore, as Mead argues, it is through the abstracted "generalized other" that the community exercises social control, and "enters as a determining factor in the individual's thinking" (p. 220).

Mead also makes an additional point about acquiring roles, in that the identification with social roles allows for the broader pattern of identifications and affiliations, such as with political parties. It is not simply that one takes the attitude of the other toward himself, but that he takes the attitudes of the other toward the broader topography of social organization. Importantly, for Mead, language plays a critical role in this process of internalization, as it serves as the "medium" through which the individual absorbs the attitudes and perspectives of the group (p. 226).

Mead does not take a firm position on why it is that children are motivated to identify with the range of roles within the broader social organization.[9] As he understands it, throughout the duration of childhood, social activity is marked by the goal of attaining affiliation and belonging. This is reflected in the various "social organizations" (p. 224) of varying degrees of permanence and importance which children are frequently creating or joining, which provide the opportunity for "playing a sort of social game" (p. 224) and the taking on of social roles. As we have mentioned, for Mead, the result of this developmental process is that the child can become a fully "self-conscious member of the community" (p. 224) through stable identification with communal attitudes and norms.

At this point, we can now revisit the question we posed at the beginning of the chapter about the development of the sensus communis. We can suggest that Mead's notion of the "generalized other" is related to Kant's notion of the sensus communis, as both Kant and Mead are referring to the incorporation of the broader perspective of the universal other into the process of thought. As such, we can suggest that Mead's theory of the self provides further developmental grounding for the emergence and crystallization of the sensus communis. Importantly, given that Mead has expressly linked the notion of "generalized other" to that of the superego, we can invoke the law of substitution, and find substantiation for our attempt establish a link between Kant and Freud; that is to say, an expanded Kantian model of reflective judgment can and should make use of the psychoanalytic concept of internalization to provide a developmental account for the emergence of the sensus communis.

Similarly, we can also revisit the question as to whether the sensus communis is contiguous with the self, or self-alien in nature. While Schafer's framework affords us one perspective, namely, that one can indeed represent the presence of the other within the self-as-place; Mead's framework offers us another approach to the question. That is to say, that for Mead there is indeed oscillation within the phenomenological experience of the self; at times, when the "me" is at the foreground of experience, one stands with the "generalized other" and regards the self from a distance. For Mead, this is a central feature of consciousness, emerging from the social origins of the self.

There is also an additional point we can make as well, related to the broader phenomenology of OCD symptomatology. Following Mead, we can suggest that within OCD, there is a heavy imbalance in the oscillation between "me" and "I"; the experience of the individual with OCD is heavily dominated by "me" against the "I." He is locked in a position of objectivity toward the self, and therefore of alienation from the self. There is little of the spontaneous activity and freedom of the "I," but an overwhelming amount of evaluation and monitoring of the self, taken as an object, by the "me."

To summarize some of the central threads of our discussion to this point, we restate briefly our response to the questions posed at the beginning of this chapter regarding the sensus communis, namely, its development as well as its integration into the structure of the self. We have proposed to consider these questions from within the framework of internalization, such that there is a transduction of norms and schemata from outside to inside the self. Following Schafer and Parsons (1958), we suggested that the process through which these become assimilated into the self and experienced as "one's own" (contiguous with the self and assimilated into the self's motivational structural such that they are not experienced as self-alien) is connected to that of superego development, which in turn is catalyzed by the processes of identification and introjection.

Our discussion of Mead has allowed us to further develop a language and framework to capture both the processes involved in internalization as well the ways in which this internalization leads to changes in the structure of the self. Specifically, while for Schafer we have discussed the ways in which fundamental conceptions of self in relation to the other (including the sense that one has "taken in" the other) shape the structure of motivation and as intrapsychic representation, Mead emphasizes the ways in which the actual substance of thought, and consciousness itself, are fundamentally dialogical. Following this characterization of thought and consciousness, we have then considered how the oscillations between subjectivity and objectivity, and specifically the ways in which the "me" may set itself up in judgment and evaluation against the spontaneity of the "I," seem to capture important components of OCD phenomenology. We turn now to Vygotsky's work on language, which also suggests that consciousness is dialogical and is the result of a process of internalization. We will then consider the implications of his theory for our discussion of OCD.

NOTES

1. Most of Mead's published work consists of lectures and papers published and edited by his students and colleagues, and published following his death. See Strauss's introduction to his volume of Mead's work for a more detailed overview of how this came about. All of the papers cited in this chapter were drawn from Strauss's anthology of selected papers (1964).

2. The elements of this response (that he must run away) are not intrinsic and automatic to the stimulus itself; rather, these elements are effectuated through access to the cultural meaning of the concept of fire. In other words, one knows to run away from a fire by tapping into the received repository of cultural knowledge.

3. To clarify, Mead is not referring here to an affective or moral empathy, but rather a more fundamental ability to represent the other in one's consciousness, across a range of functions.

4. In this essay, Mead actually refers to it as a "ditch," while in Mind, Self, and Society, Mead uses the word "chasm" as part of his more expansive description. To keep things consistent, we use only the word "chasm." See below.

5. It is beyond the scope of the discussion to provide an analysis of Mead's conception here of animal consciousness and psychology, as the central points of his model stand on their own.

6. See footnote on p. 205 where Mead acknowledges that the essential concept of "taking the attitude of the other" is "generally recognized," but argues that in his model, this form of "social intelligence" is "not merely one of the various aspects or expressions of intelligence or of intelligent behavior, but is the very essence of its character."

7. To our understanding, Mead's account does not diminish the self's freedom or agency, and one still retains full control over their will and their freedom of choice even while acting as the "I." Rather, Mead seems to be suggesting that "me" and "I" are both continually present in a sense of alternating between foreground and background. That is, one may have an idea about doing something (formulated in the preceding "me" phase), but this idea is more of an intention, and has a degree of abstraction vis a vis the specific contours of the situation itself. Accordingly, in the process of carrying out the idea from intention to fully-realized action, one firsts formulates a plan and then attempts to carry it out (the "I" phase). In the phase (and moments of) of action ("I"), one's attention and focus are on the process of "doing," and there is then a decreased sense of self-consciousness and reflexive evaluation.

However, there is still a constant and ongoing process of evaluation and readjustment as one acts, in order to determine whether the given actions have resulted in the intended effects in the world around him. For instance, one can choose to tell a joke ("me"), and in the process of telling realize that it would be better not to tell it as he had planned. Thus, in the process of action ("I") there is then ongoing evaluation and readjustment ("me").

8. See p. 238 where Mead explicitly references Freud and the Freudian concept of the "censor," by which he means the superego.

9. Mead does not really take up the larger question of motivation (either conscious or unconscious), and does not consider why it is that someone might be drawn to any given social role over any other possibility, e.g., why might one boy identify with firemen while another might identify with a politician. As we shall see, Vygotsky does in fact invoke the "motivating sphere of consciousness" (p. 107), though he too does not elaborate.

Chapter 4

Internalization and the Social Origins of Consciousness in Vygotsky's Model of the Self

Vygotsky's work on language shares many similarities with Mead's,[1] and offers a complementary perspective on the processes of internalization and the development of the self. Vygotsky's account is important to our discussion because it allows us to revisit the internalization of the role played by others, outside of the self, in the guidance, organization, and direction of the child's behavior. Additionally, it allows us to further consider the particular features of consciousness that, rooted in the social development of the self, generate oscillations between self-contiguous and self-alien modes of subjective experience. We commence then with a brief overview of Vygotsky's treatment of these themes. Our account draws primarily from three papers[2]; the first is his paper Dynamics and Structure of the Adolescent (2004), the second is Genesis of Higher Mental Functions (1997), and lastly, his famous treatise on the nature of speech, Thought and Word (2004).

Vygotsky, in his paper Dynamics and Structure of the Adolescent (2004), takes the maximalist position that *all* higher mental functions have their origins in social relationships which have been internalized. As Vygotsky explains[3]:

> every function in the cultural development of the child appears on the stage twice, in two forms—at first as social, then as psychological; at first as a form of cooperation between people, as a group, an intermental category, then as a means of individual behavior, as an intramental category. This is the general law for the construction of all higher mental functions. (pp. 473–474)

That is to say, Vygotsky asserts a fundamental continuity between interpersonal and intrapsychic functioning, such that the individual replicates in his own reflexive conduct what he does in the social sphere. This continuity is the result of a process of internalization:

Thus, the structures of higher mental functions represent a cast of collective social relations between people. These structures are nothing other than a transfer into the personality of an inward relation of a social order that constitutes the basis of the social structure of the human personality. The personality is by nature social. (p. 474)

Accordingly, Vygotsky, (following Janet), takes the position that the structure of speech itself reflects its origins within the social world. More specifically, "the word is a command" (p. 473), in the sense that one uses language in their attempts to shape and direct (or even compel) the behaviors of others around them. Eventually, this regulatory function of language is expressed reflexively, toward oneself. Language toward oneself becomes the primary tool for regulating one's own behavior. As we will see, this is connected to the interaction between language and thought, and to the internalization of external speech.

In his paper Genesis of Higher Mental Functions,[4] Vygotsky, again following Janet, presents the same trajectory:

In general, we could say that the relations between higher mental functions were at one time real relations between people. I relate to myself in the same way that people relate to me. As verbal thinking represents an internalization of speech . . . . The original psychology of the function of the word is a social function. . . (p. 103)

Regulating another's behavior by means of the word leads gradually to the development of verbalized behavior of the individual himself. (p. 104)

That is to say, speech, at its core, has an interpersonal function, and serves a regulatory function within social existence; it is an attempt to bring about a change in the behavior of another. It is this regulatory function which becomes internalized, such that speech becomes a means for reflexive, intra-psychic regulation and organization of one's own behavior. For Vygotsky,[5] this reflexive regulatory function is ultimately performed by thought, which he characterizes as a form of reflexive communication within the self; thought is in essence "inner speech," defined more clearly as "speech for oneself" (2004, p. 80). We turn then to Vygotsky's analysis of the connection between language and thought, presented in his paper Thought and Word (2004).

Accordingly, Vygotsky's analysis is based on two central points. The first point is that the use of language in social communication and its use in language-based thought reflect an underlying "unity" (2004, p. 66); speech follows a developmental trajectory, in which the distinctions between the two functions of speech (inner and outer speech) emerge from a common point of origin. In order to substantiate the presence of this developmental process, Vygotsky focuses on the particular qualities of "egocentric speech," and identifies this form of speech as the transition point in development; the differentiation between the two functions of speech has begun to emerge, but full differentiation has not yet happened.

The second point, relatedly, is Vygotsky's contention about the nature of "word meaning" (p. 66). For Vygotsky, speech serves a function, which is to communicate something meaningful to someone; as such, any analysis of speech must also take into account the meaning of the word, as this constitutes the intention of the communicative act. Similarly, the meaning of a word is essentially "a concept" (p. 66), which for Vygotsky is a "psychological" (p. 66) representation; in turn, the representation and generation of conceptual material constitutes "an act of thought" (p. 66). Accordingly, "word meaning" then is the synthesis of two processes, those of language and thought; and it is this "unit" (see p. 66) of analysis which clarifies the fundamental connection between inner and social speech.

We present here our reconstruction of Vygotsky's argument, beginning with his discussion of egocentric speech in young children. In the basic parameters of the phenomenon, Vygotsky accepts the general findings of Piaget's research. Specifically, there are three features of egocentric speech which Vygotsky addresses in his paper, and which he attributes to Piaget's observations. The first of these findings is that egocentric speech "has the character of external speech" (p. 87). That is to say, when the child talks to themselves, they sound to an observer as if they are talking to someone else.

The second point is that "egocentric speech is a collective monologue" (p. 87); children tend to talk to themselves in this way when they are playing with other children, but not when they are by themselves. Vygotsky, citing Grünbaum, describes Grünbaum's observations and characterization of this "collective monologue." Vygotsky notes that though the children playing together in a group seem to be talking to each other, such that a running transcript "looks like conversation" (p. 87), each child is in reality only talking to themselves; closer attention to the sequence of comments indicates that the children do not in fact "respond to one another" (p. 87).

And lastly, Vygotsky relates the observation that children's egocentric speech "is accompanied by an illusion of understanding" (p. 87). As Vygotsky explains, "the child believes and assumes that the egocentric expressions that he addresses to no one are understood by those around him" (p. 87).

This last point serves as a "point of departure" (p. 81) for Vygotsky's analysis, as the central issue that defines Vygotsky's approach to egocentric speech is his disagreement with Piaget's characterization of its essential character and function. For Piaget, egocentric speech emerges from the child's fundamental egocentrism and his insufficient relatedness to the social world around him; the child is fundamentally "immersed in himself" (p. 87).[6] He talks out loud, to himself, expecting others magically to understand what he is saying without going through the process of taking into account the pragmatics of communication. In essence, the child is not capable of meaningful perspective-taking, and cannot yet construct a coherent theory of mind. As such, the child maintains a sense of his own relatedness to the world (reflected in the "illusion of understanding" present during egocentric speech), though the actual quality of this relatedness is so degraded and nebulous that the child cannot really be said to be meaningfully connected.

To Vygotsky's understanding, Piaget's analysis of egocentric speech is rooted in his theory of the child's broader egocentrism. Accordingly (again, to his understanding of Piaget's position), the "illusion of understanding" is not a precondition for the child's egocentric speech, but rather an artifact of his "insufficient socialization." (p. 82). The child feels some impulse to communicate something to those around him, but is not really capable of doing so in any kind of consistent manner. Thus, his speech is not really intelligible to those around him, and he does not take into account the responses (or lack thereof) of his audience to his words. As the child's theory of mind develops to the point where genuine perspective-taking has developed, egocentric speech disappears, and is replaced by fully understandable social communication.

However, Vygotsky, again following Grünbaum, takes issue with this characterization. He references a series of experiments in which children's egocentric talk significantly decreases under conditions in which the child is no longer able to maintain the "illusion of understanding," such as when the child perceives interpersonal communication to be impossible or fruitless. Among these experimental conditions, a child was surrounded by other children who were either hearing-impaired, or who speak a foreign language; or was moved away from the larger group of other children, and so on. The level of egocentric speech was observed to drop significantly under these conditions. Vygotsky argues that according to Piaget, who emphasizes the character of the child's fundamental egocentrism, we would expect these conditions to have no effect on children's egocentric speech, since the child's fundamental orientation is anyway egocentric even within close proximity to other children.

Rather, Vygotsky argues that the findings of these studies support the position expressed by Grünbaum, that the "illusion of understanding" is actually a critical condition for the child's egocentric speech. In fact, it actually speaks to the essential "social connectedness of the child's mind" (p. 87). Vygotsky explains further the significance of the "illusion of understanding" in Grünbaum's position. That is, for Vygotsky (following Grünbaum), the phenomenon of egocentric speech is linked to the nature of consciousness and its development; consciousness itself begins as a *collective* consciousness[7] in which "the thoughts of each are the common property of all" (p. 87), and follows a trajectory of increased individuation. Ultimately, it reaches the form of an individual and private consciousness. It is this same trajectory that is present in speech, where a process that is initially a social one becomes progressively internalized, until it crystallizes as language-based thought. Egocentric speech is a midpoint in this process, and "demonstrates the inadequate differentiation of the child's individual mind from the social whole" (p. 86). As Vygotsky further explains:

> this transition constitutes the general law of the development of all higher mental functions. (p. 82)

Here, Vygotsky references his paper "The Development of Higher Mental Functions"[8], and the "general law" of the development of these functions. This is an important point, and one which we will return to shortly.

More specifically, for Vygotsky, egocentric speech emerges from an increased internalization of speech function, but within the matrix of an insufficiently differentiated collective consciousness. Thus, egocentric speech serves a specific function; it "facilitates intellectual orientation, conscious awareness, the overcoming of difficulties and impediments, and imagination and thinking" (p. 83). As Vygotsky makes clear, this function "is closely related to the function of inner speech" (p. 82), and therefore represents a transition point in the process of internalizing a guiding and facilitative function, initially present in the social world, and eventually reconstituted in the intrapsychic world.

Since Vygotsky himself references his earlier paper, it seems indicated to connect his characterization of the function of egocentric speech as presented in Thought and Word to his exposition of Janet's position in Genesis of Higher Mental Functions, in order to present a more fully integrated model of the internalization of speech (see again note 4, below). Accordingly, the following model emerges from these two papers: the origin of speech lies in the social world, as the child's means of regulating the behavior of those around him in order to attain what he needs. Subsequently, this mode of regulation is then used by the child to regulate and direct his own behavior through the use of language, in reflexive communication and as "speech for oneself". When this internalization of language use is complete, there is a clear distinction between "speech for oneself," which is inner speech, and "speech for others" (p. 82), which is external speech. Prior to the completion of this process, the distinction is not as clear, since consciousness itself has not been fully individuated, and thus, based on the "illusion of understanding," speech for oneself is not private, but rather takes place within the matrix of a shared social consciousness. As such, egocentric speech reflects the beginnings of guiding and directing one's own behavior, and the beginnings of an individuation of consciousness; nonetheless, consciousness remains within the matrix of the larger social world, thereby perpetuating the child's "illusion of understanding," which in turn gives rise to a form of speech that is at the same time for oneself yet shared with others.

On the basis of his analysis, Vygotsky returns to consider some of the central elements of the structures of inner speech, and some important structural distinctions between thought and speech.

The first of these points concerns a term Vygotsky calls "predicativity" (p. 91). For Vygotsky, there can exist a disjunction between "psychological and grammatical subject and predicate" (p. 74); more specifically, Vygotsky defines the "psychological subject" of a sentence as the element which is represented first in consciousness, the object with which the mind is concerned, such that the rest of the statement will refer to that object. This does not always correspond to the grammatical subject. Vygotsky considers the following example, using the sentence "the clock fell":

> "I am working at my desk. I hear a noise from a falling object and ask what it was that fell. The same phrase is used ["the clock fell"] to answer my question, but here it is the falling that is initially represented in consciousness. "Fell" is what is spoken about in this phrase; it is the psychological subject. The clock is what is said of this subject, what arises in consciousness second; it is the psychological predicate. This thought might better be expressed as follows: "What fell is the clock." (p. 75)

Using this distinction, Vygotsky analyzes the (psychological) syntax of inner speech, and argues that it is marked by "pure and absolute predicativity" (p. 91), in which the psychological subject of the phrase is left out, though "present in the interlocutor's thoughts" (p. 91); that is to say, the subject is by definition always known to and represented by the thinker himself.

Vygotsky provides the following illustration of "pure predicativity": he describes a group of people waiting for "the B tram" (p. 91). One of them sees the tram approaching, and calls out "It's coming." There is no need to spell out what exactly is coming, or what it will do for them now that it has arrived, or where it will take them; these concepts are already fully represented and fully present in the thought of each passenger. Similarly, in inner speech, the thinker already represents in his thoughts the subject around which further thought will unfold. The inner speech which takes place in reference to the given subject does not need to include any words explicitly referencing the subject, since it is by definition already represented in the consciousness of thinker, with all its nuances and colorations, the moment he begins to think about it.

Thus, for Vygotsky, inner speech represents an "inner dialogue" (p. 97) of reflexive communication, in which there are two parties to the conversation; the speaker and the "interlocutor" (p. 91). who are both present in consciousness. Vygotsky contrasts this element of inner speech (p. 94) with the syntax of written word. In the process of writing, there can be no "illusion of understanding"; the writer recognizes that his reader will have no knowledge of a shared implicit subject of expression, and no "shared common subject in thought" (p. 96). Writing is therefore "speech without an interlocutor" (p. 94), and consequently, it must be the most precise, articulated, and elongated form of speech. Everything that is implicit in the writer's mind must be made explicit in text for it to be intelligible to the reader.

Similarly, oral speech can also fall along a continuum. Sometimes, a shared understanding can be justifiably presumed, as in Vygotsky's example of the B tram. In these situations, dialogue will typically be truncated, since so much is jointly presumed and represented simultaneously in the minds of talker and interlocutor. At other times, the speaker will have to be more expansive and articulate, or risk being misunderstood.

Accordingly, Vygotsky argues that egocentric speech, in this sense, is similar to inner speech; the "illusion of understanding," a product of a shared communal consciousness, leads the child to presume that the subject of his speech (and all else that is implicit but unexpressed in his own mind) is simultaneously represented in the consciousness of his interlocutors. Thus, the child's egocentric speech[9] is similarly characterized by its brevity, its predicativity (reflected in the absence of a clear subject), and its consequent unintelligibility to the interlocutor.

Relatedly, Vygotsky introduces another concept, which he refers to as "word sense"; he provides the following definition:

a word's sense is the aggregate of all the psychological facts that arise in our consciousness as a result of the word. (p. 100)

Word sense, then, includes the affective and associative (or resonant) elements of the word, which are conjured and stimulated by the word, and which transcend a definite meaning "identical in all contexts" (p. 100). Vygotsky provides the example of referencing the titles of famous literary works, which conjures the drama and meaning of the whole book through the use of a single phrase, such as "Hamlet."

Accordingly, Vygotsky considers this element of word sense in relation the dialects of specific social groups. He explains that dialects are a function of word sense, whereby words begin take on "different colorations" and "sense nuances" (p. 103) grasped fully only by the members of the group.

Vygtsoky maintains that inner speech is also marked by this sense of "dialect." The particular networks of meanings and associations represented by the single word are known only by the thinker himself, and these networks cannot be fully conveyed to others by the external expression (through language) of this single word. As Vygotsky explains further, the task of conveying meaning to others requires the "restructuring of speech" (p. 104), leading to a different structure and syntax, expressed in external speech.

Essentially, then, for Vygotsky, as we have said, inner speech is an internal dialogue of reflexive communication. Its syntax is marked by its predicativity, and by its brevity, which is also a result of one's access to his own idiosyncratic database of the "senses" conveyed and conjured by his words. In the broader sense, we can say that the thinker "knows what he means," and that he alone has the most privileged access to the meaning of his own thoughts. We will return to this point shortly, for it is critical for the conclusion of Vygotsky's analysis.

We can add an additional point here as well. If we further follow the connection between the two papers, made by Vygotsky himself, the following emerges: that even in thought, there is a part of self that is directing (the commanding function performed by the "speaker"), and a part that is being directed (the receptive "interlocutor"). We will return to this point as well in the course of our discussion of the implications of Vygotsky's model for explicating the broader phenomenology of OCD compulsions.

Vygotsky argues that despite the connections between thought and speech which he has suggested (reflected in inner speech), it cannot be said that thought and speech are identical. Rather, thought constitutes an independent plane of intellectual functioning, distinct from speech and communication:

> Thought is characterized by a movement, an unfolding. It establishes a relationship between one thing and another. In a word, thought fulfills some function. It resolves some task. Thought's flow and movement does not correspond directly with the unfolding of speech . . . The two processes manifest a unity but not an identity. (p. 105)

Vygotsky provides two illustrations of this distinction. First, he distinguishes between the simple meaning of a phrase, and the broader functional role the phrase is intended to play. Vygotsky provides the following example, with the familiar phrase "the clock fell": suppose that there are two people in a room, and one person asks another, "why has the clock stopped?," and the other one answers "the clock fell." It is quite plausible that in addition to providing a concrete explanation for what has caused the clock to stop working (damage due to the fall), the answer also is intended to communicate that "it is not my fault," the clock fell on its own. As Vygotsky explains further, this thought (that "it's not my fault") could be expressed in entirely different words without even mentioning the clock explicitly. For Vygotsky, this demonstrates that one can distinguish between the functional and the semantic meanings of the phrase, which explains as well why the functional meaning of a thought can be expressed in many different syntactical forms.

Additionally, this distinction results in differential representations in consciousness. The functional meaning of a phrase, the expression of its purpose, is represented in the mind as a "whole" (p. 106); all the words that are a part of this phrase are represented in the mind "simultaneously" (p. 106). Thus, the thought "it is not my fault" is represented as a full unit, even before the formulation of the particular phrase (and the selection of particular words) which will ultimately be expressed as external speech. Vygotsky expresses then the following observation about the nature of the relationship between thought and speech:

> Thought is always something whole, something with significantly greater extent and volume than the individual word. . . . *What is contained simultaneously in thought unfolds sequentially in speech.* Thought can be compared to a hovering cloud which gushes a shower of words. (p. 106)

Vygotsky argues further, that, thought, in its purest form, contains meaning without words at all. He suggests that while every thought has a meaning, not every thought has words; meaning to say, one cannot always access and articulate the meaning of one's thoughts. Doing so requires an active process of converting "background" (p. 106) meanings, nuances, and colorations into language, which is not always successful. For Vygotsky, these difficulties are reflected in the phenomenon when one finds themselves unable to put their thoughts into words.

Vygotsky suggests that there is then a process in which meaning is accessed and transformed into speech: first, meaning is instantiated in the language-based thought of inner speech (for oneself), and then it can be further transformed into external speech for others. Language then is the medium through which the function of pure thought interacts with the function of speech and communication.

Having established that thought, is independent of language, Vygotsky attempts to suggest how it is that thoughts themselves emerge. For Vygotsky, the ultimate source of thought is in the "motivating sphere of consciousness":

> Thought has its origins in the motivating sphere of consciousness, a sphere that includes our inclinations and needs, our interests and impulses, and our affect and emotion.[10] (p. 107)

That is to say, the function of thought (that is, pure thought) is to make possible the expression of feeling and the realization of motivation. It can be said then, that for Vygotsky, the process of accessing and interpreting the meaning of thought is ultimately a process of discerning what one feels and what one desires. Similarly, to fully understand the thinking of someone else requires an understanding of their "affective volitional basis" (p. 107).

There are then two points about Vygotsky's analysis which we can make at this juncture. The first of these points concerns Vygotsky's thesis, following Janet (see note 4, below), that language-based thought should be understood as the self reflexively guiding and directing its own behavior, and that it emerges through the internalization of a social process. This aspect of Vygotsky's theory is connected to the idea we suggested following our presentation of Schafer's model of internalization, that, following Shapiro, there is indeed a "directing" or "guiding" function performed by the child's caregivers. For Vygotsky, it is the development of the child's ability to regulate the other (through language) which is then broadened into the regulation of the self, whereas for Shapiro it is the guidance and regulation of the other which is internalized. However, they both locate the emergence of the child's capacity for self-direction and self-guidance within the social sphere, and characterize it as the internalization of an external process. In a sense, then, Vygotsky's model offers at least a partial confirmation for our suggestion; that this function is a distinct one, that it plays an important role in the child's psychological development, and that can be said to be internalized.

However, that being, said, there is an important element absent from Vygotsky's presentation, one which is critical for our discussion. We have suggested earlier[11] that the process of taking over these functions is not merely cognitive, but also affective and representational; that is to say, following Schafer, the process of internalization is both mediated by and results in changes in representations of the self, important others, and the self "in relation" to others. These changes in representation occur both in the nature of the representations themselves, as well as in the intrapsychic location of these representations. Thus, the process of taking over the "guiding" functions involves the process of identification, in which the child actually comes to see themselves like (and therefore as) the parent, in the sense of having assumed not just their function, but also their qualities.

We have suggested then, that what is central to the process of the child's assumption of the parental "guiding function" is how the child orients themselves to this function, within the context of the relationship to the parent. For instance, a rebellious child who is unwilling to direct their own behavior with any meaningful reference to the expectations of his environment, likely bears the attitude that these demands, and the people who make them, are completely (or mostly) external to him; they have not become incorporated into his motivational structure, as Schafer would say. Superego development, at the other end, implies that the child bears the attitude that the expectations that others have of him are also his own.

Similarly, for Shapiro, the acceptance of parental authority is rooted in the emergence of a specific orientation toward the parent and toward the self. It implies an object-relation with beliefs and attitudes toward the parent, and second-order attitudes toward one's own impulses. Accepting the parental authority is not simply a question of why, in given moment x, does a child listen to parent y? For that can be for any number of reasons, including the fear of punishment. Rather, Shapiro is describing a way in which the child, in his recognition of the parent's understanding of the world, endows the parental figure with certain qualities; their knowledge, their competence, and so on. As such, we can say that for Shapiro, what it means to say that a parent has become an authority for the child is to say that the child, in his object-representations of the parent, endows the parent's judgments and directives with an **a priori** legitimacy. There is a sense that the parent is the one to turn to when in doubt, that they are the arbiter of right and wrong, good and bad, and that they "know" the right way to do things. Concurrently, the child modifies, to a large degree, his own self-representation; he restrains his own impulses, and subordinates his own "sense of things" to that of the adult. He defers to the authority and judgment of the adult.

Accordingly, within the context of chronic indecisiveness and compulsive doubting, we have suggested that what is at stake is not merely a cognitive or metacognitive issue. Rather, it is a question of one's own orientation to the "determining function" that he must "take over" from the parental figure, and fulfill for himself. The adult, in fulfilling the "guiding" function for the child, also provides a determining function for the child. That is to say, in the natural course of events, the child experiences states of uncertainty. These states can emerge from within the child, in the sense of not knowing how to do something, and from without; the child recognizes the adult's authority, and understands that he must accommodate his impulses to the expectations and directions of others. As such, while awaiting the directives and instruction of the parent (and in some instances having subordinated his own "sense of things" in those moments), the child then enters a state of not knowing what to do, in the sense of determining the correct (in instances of practical uncertainty) or approved and sanctioned course of action. In states of both pragmatic and normative uncertainties, the child looks to the parent to resolve the uncertainty for them, to *determine* for them what to do. This function, too, must eventually be taken over by the child.

As we have suggested, this too should be mediated by the processes of internalization and identification; the child comes to trust their own ability to resolve their doubts, render judgments, and make determinations because they come to see themselves as possessing the same (or sufficient) requisite qualities and qualifications for performing these functions as their parents possess. For instance, a child recognizes that there are some decisions they can make themselves, and others which need to be made by their parents; for instance, they can "feel" mature enough, or intelligent enough, to make one decision, but recognize the gap between themselves and the parent in the degree of these qualities, such that decisions which require more maturity or more intelligence should be made by those with "more maturity" or "more intelligence." At different stages of this process of "taking over," a child comes to feel that they "know what to do," which would seem to emerge from the child's sense that their perceptions and interpretations of reality, and their own determinations, reliably and sufficiently overlap with those of the parental figure. In short, they come to see making these kinds of decisions and determinations as something "which they do."

In those whose experience of uncertainty is chronic and pervasive, we have suggested that this "determining" function remains outsourced to others; it is not something the child came to see as something that they themselves "do," but remained for the child something which ought to be done by others. Thus, the child bears the attitude, regarding his own ability to decide, to judge, and to determine, that he is not the final authority; he does not accord his own impulses and interpretations with an a priori legitimacy. Rather, there is always "someone" else to whom it is either more prudent, or critically necessary, to whom to turn. This "other" is endowed with a high degree of some quality that is prized and desired, and thought of as necessary for "knowing." The "other" understands better, discerns better, is wiser, remembers better, or something to that effect. We have attempted to show how this schematic representation of a mediating role of the parental authority (and the child's representations of self and other within the context of the relationship with the adults who performed this function for him) between the resolution of the child's uncertainty and definitive "knowing" of what is correct maps on to the theory proposed by Lazarov et al. (2010) about the need for "proxies" in the attainment of knowledge.

Vygotsky, however, does not in these papers make clear reference to the role of attitude in the process of acquiring and internalizing external functions. Nor does he center his account on changes in self-representation. In other words, Vygotsky's model of internalization overlaps partially with Schafer's discussion (and Hartmann's inclusion of the term) of the way functions are "taken over" or "taken in." However, Vygotsky does not integrate the issue of object-representation (much less object-relations) into his account of development.

The second point, emerging from Vygotsky's formulation of the function of egocentric and internal speech, concerns the broader phenomenology of compulsions within OCD. For Vygotsky, as for Mead, thought is an inner dialogue of reflexive communication. For Mead, thought involves alternating between the poles of self as subject and self as object. Similarly, for Vygotsky, thought involves the reflexive communication of the self guiding and directing its own behavior. Moreover, for Vygotsky, there also seem to be two polarities within the self;[12] that part which serves the commanding function,[13] and that of the "interlocutor"; the part which expresses the "motivating" sphere of consciousness (and thereby conveys the drive), and the part which interprets the thought (as the drive-derivative) and attempts to actualize it.

As we suggested in our discussion of Mead, this account seems to provide a fuller description of OCD compulsions. In Vygotsky's formulation, we can say that compulsions represent the dominance of the commanding function over that of the "interlocutor." One part of the mind is perpetually attempting to compel behavior (and regulate behavior), and the other part of the mind is in a perpetual state of feeling compelled. Importantly, within the phenomenology of compulsions, the part of the self which is compelling is felt to be self-alien, whereas the self is felt to be more closely aligned with the parts of the mind which are being compelled. In our discussion of Mead we suggested that this can be understood from an object-relational framework, in the sense of reenactment and repetition of roles and states experienced in relation to adult authority figures, and perhaps even indicating the presence of an introject.

By linking thought and motivation, Vygotsky's formulation offers us the opportunity to explore a different aspect of this phenomenology, and revisit a question we have posed a number of times in this work. More specifically, if thought arises from within the "motivating sphere of consciousness," what does it mean to say that there is an expressed motivation (i.e., the compulsive thought) which is experienced as self-alien, and deriving from outside the parts of the mind which feel self-contiguous? Again, while our previous discussions have centered on various elements of the processes of internalization, we can highlight another aspect of the emerging self which will allow us to tie together some of the various threads which have been suggested to this point. To do so, we will look to the writings of Winnicott which suggest the processes through which the self emerges either as energized by or alienated from its own "motivating sphere of consciousness" (in Vygotsky's language) and the impulses which animate it.

NOTES

1. See for instance Edwards's (2007) chapter in the Cambridge Companion to Vygotsky comparing the two theorists, as well as articles by Koczanowitz (1994) and Glock (1986).

2. In this book, citations from the papers Dynamics and Structure of the Adolescent as well as Thought and Word are from Rieber and Robinson's *The Essential Vygotsky* (2004). These papers were reprinted from the published six-volume English translation of Vygotsky's writings, *The Collected Works of L.S. Vygotsky* (1987-1999), edited by Rieber. The citation from Genesis of Higher Mental Functions is from Volume 4 of the *Collected Works*.

3. Vyogtsky's own articulation of these points is very strong; accordingly, we provide here portions of his own writing. Additionally, of the first two papers, we find his writing in this paper to be the most expansive and clear, so we begin our presentation with his paper on adolescence. We note as well that our intention is to consider here the implications of Vygotsky's broader framework and its focus on internalization, especially in connection to the development of thought. Accordingly, our account is not tethered to the specifically maximalist positions as he has articulated them.

4. We reference this paper here as well because Vygotsky refers to this paper in Word and Speech, and his cross-referencing is important because it allows us to more fully reconstruct his model. Note that in this paper, Vygotsky is more equivocal about the specifics of Janet's theory (though he seems to accept Janet's more general paradigm about the internalization of speech), but in his paper on adolescence, Vygotsky more clearly follows Janet's position that language has a regulatory function; it therefore seems appropriate to suggest a link between Vygotsky's position in Thought and Word and Janet's position about the regulatory function of speech.

5. In this, we follow Berk (1984), who identifies *regulation* as the function of private speech in Thought and Word; in this, she connects these two papers. Though this is not explicitly stated in Thought and Word, it seems to be alluded to by Vygotsky's own cross-referencing, as we will describe below. Berk is most clear on pp. 271–272, that "private speech was seen as thought spoken by the child out loud, and its purpose was to communicate with the self for self-guidance and self-direction", which strongly supports this reading.

6. We present here Piaget's position as summarized by Vygotsky, who follows and presents Grünbaum's summary of Piaget in contrast with his own.

7. This emphasis on the collective origins of consciousness may be seen in connection to Vygotsky's efforts to formulate a Marxist psychology (see Packer, 2018, for a more recent overview of Vygotsky's connection to Marx).

8. This identification follows that of the editor's note.

9. Vygotsky notes that as the child matures, his egocentric speech becomes less abbreviated, and fuller; as the "illusion" wears off, his speech for others begins to take the same structure as it does for adults.

10. See Wilson and Weinstein (1992) for a discussion of how Vygotsky's brief formulation here suggests a potential synthesis with psychoanalytic drive theory.

11. For the purposes of clarifying this point, we provide here a brief restatement of our thesis.

12. In fact, at the conclusion of Thought and Word, Vygotsky strongly implies that the structure of consciousness itself is dialogical in nature. Referencing Feuerbach, he writes that words are "absolutely impossible for one person but possible for two" (p. 110).

13. Based on the proposed integration of Janet's theory of language and that of Vygotsky.

Chapter 5

Self-Near and Self-Alien Elements of Personality within Winnicott's Model of Psychological Development

We now turn our attention to Winnicott, and provide an outline of his account of the development of the self. In particular, we will focus on his analysis of how it is that the self endows the external world with meaning and vitality. We begin first with a discussion of Winnicott's conceptualization of the emergence of the self during infancy,[1] and then provide an overview of two papers, Transitional Objects and Transitional Phenomena (1953), and his paper Ego Distortion in Terms of True and False Self (1965).[2] For Winnicott, the period of infancy is broadly characterized by a transition from a state of merger to one of individuation as it passes through a series of stages of maternal care. As Winnicott famously writes, "'There is no such thing as an infant,' meaning, of course, that whenever one finds an infant one finds maternal care, and without maternal care there would be no infant" (1960, p. 587). Initially, the child's ego is exceedingly weak, and requires the strength and support of the maternal ego in order to both organize and meet its physiological and psychological needs. Yet through the mother's devoted and attentive care, the infant's ego is sufficiently strengthened such that it can function independently:

> the infant ego eventually becomes free of the mother's ego support, so that the
> infant achieves mental detachment from the mother, that is, differentiation into
> a separate personal self. (1960, p. 587)

As mentioned, Winnicott identifies a series of paradigms or modes, which comprise the mother's pattern of care for the infant. These are "the holding phase," followed by "mother and infant living together," and then "father, mother, and infant, all three living together." In the "holding phase," the mother's consistently empathic attunement to the child's needs creates a "total environment" (1960, p. 588) of a "routine of care" (1960, p. 591) in which the infant is protected from overwhelming and painful sensory exposure as well as from sustained and prolonged deprivation of physiological needs. Importantly, Winnicott considers the infant to be "merged" (1960, p. 588) with the mother during this stage. We will return soon to describe this phase more fully, as it occupies an important place in Winnicott's developmental theory of the self. In the two "living with" stages, the infant transitions more clearly from merger to object-relatedness (first to the mother, and subsequently to father) as the infant begins to differentiate between "me" and "not-me."

Returning to the "holding phase," we mention here some of the critical processes which take place during this stage of the mother-infant relationship. For Winnicott, the central achievement of this stage is a consolidation of a "continuity of being" (1960, p. 590), during which the infant builds up both a coherent rendering of his environment as well as an embodied sense of self by integrating sensory inputs (sights, sounds, smells), internal needs (such as hunger, or the desire to be held), and bodily sensations into meaningful schemata. Winnicott refers to this embodied self as "psyche indwelling in the soma" (1960, p. 589), and it emerges from "a linkage of motor and sensory and functional experiences with the infant's new state of being a person" (1960, p. 589). For instance, the infant begins to link their own experience of hunger with a specific set of bodily sensations, behavioral responses (such as crying and screaming), indications of the mother's presence (such as her voice), and then followed by the experience of being fed.

Importantly, it is this process of early schematization which marks the beginnings of the infant's construction of a reality which is stable and organized, and scaffolds the emergence of the infant's ego and sense of self. It is this process which allows the infant to "make sense" of what is happening both to him and within him.

Winnicott (1960) explains that this process of integrating disparate environmental and somatic elements into a program of expectations and meanings is facilitated by the mother's caretaking, and especially by her ability to provide regular, dependable care for the infant. It is especially through the establishment of empathically attuned caretaking routines that the infant can begin to assemble these sensory-somatic schemata and can begin to comfortably develop this sense of "indwelling" in soma.

Relatedly, Winnicott suggests that the development of this "psychosomatic indwelling" leads to the infant's earliest experience of the boundary between "me" and "not-me," which is through the infant's ability to differentiate between somatic experience located within the body and sensory input through the skin:

As a further development there comes into existence what might be called a limiting membrane, which to some extent (in health) is equated with the surface of the skin, and has a position between the infant's "me" and his "not-me." So the infant comes to have an inside and an outside, and a body-scheme. In this way meaning comes to the function of intake and output; moreover, it gradually becomes meaningful to postulate a personal or inner psychic reality for the infant. (1960, p. 589)

Accordingly, for Winnicott, the achievement of these processes marks the conclusion of the "holding phase" and lead to the emergence of a self, whereby "the infant becomes a person, an individual in his own right" (1960, p. 589).[3] This then allows the infant to transition to the phase of "living with" and object-relations, during which the infant transitions from a state of "merger" with the mother to one in which it comes to regard her as a separate entity.

For Winnicott, the unfolding of this process from merger to separation is critically important, since it must be accomplished in a way that does not threaten or destroy the infant's "continuity of being." Within this context, it is necessary to mention here Winnicott's notion of x+y+z time (1971). Specifically, Winnicott argues that the process of separation is accomplished successfully when the infant can enter a transitional phase (between merger and separation) in which it can symbolically represent the mother's presence even in her absence. This takes place on two levels: the first is through the identification of the "transitional object" (p. 96), onto which the symbolism of the mother is projected and in which this symbolism is instantiated[4]; and the second is within the infant's own mind, such that the infant is able to retain and conjure the "imago" (1971, p. 97) of the mother even when she is no longer present, and which provides the infant with a continued sense of wholeness and wellbeing. Thus, for Winnicott, separation is almost paradoxical, in that it is essentially a continuation of the original relationship with the mother; just now, the mother's presence has become internalized.

However, Winnicott argues that this capacity for mental representation of the maternal imago is nonetheless limited, to a significant degree, by the infant's experience of the mother's actual presence. An infant may retain an inner sense of connectedness to the mother when she has moved a few feet away but is still present within the room, but may lose this sense of connectedness when she leaves the room. As Winnicott explains, the infant's capacity to "hold on" to the sense of the mother's presence is a result of a continued "reinforcement" (1971, p. 97) of her presence; the infant might continue to hear her voice, or see her still within the room. Without this reinforcement, the maternal "imago" recedes from the infant's consciousness, and the infant is left with a terrifying sense of aloneness and disintegration. Winnicott represents this temporally: the maternal imago can linger in the infant's mind for *x* time, after which the infant can no longer represent the mother's presence, and begins to feel alone. Should the mother come back within (as experienced by the infant) a certain short period of time *y*, the infant may be reassured easily by the mother's return, and the few moments of aloneness will not have fundamentally altered the infant's experience of the world. Indeed it is this brief aloneness that provides the infant the experience of being separate in an expansive sense. However, anything beyond *y* moments (meaning *y* + *z* moments) is beyond the ego's tolerance for distress, and will therefore leave the infant with a sense that their experience of the rhythms of life has been fundamentally shaken and altered.

Having laid out Winnicott's thinking about the emergence of the self, we now turn our attention to his account of the essential activity and functioning of the self. In his paper on transitional objects, Winnicott (1953) takes as the focus of his study the process through which little children become attached to a favorite toy or doll or blanket, which seemingly serves the function of comforting them when they are upset or when they are lonely. Winnicott suggests that these objects are "transitional" in the sense that they are not experienced by the infant as a part of the body, but are not yet understood as belonging to external reality. Rather, they are a concretization and a crystallization of a meaningful and comforting mode of being and experiencing; in this instance, the infant's closeness to its mother. The infant is aware that the object is not the mother, yet is nonetheless able to experience it as possessing a "real" vitality and a meaning that approximates "mother" or "comfort" or "closeness."

Essentially then, the meaning of the transitional object is not one which is objective, but rather one which is subjective; it is endowed with a given meaning by a given person. Winnicott explains that this phenomenon is rooted in one of the central tasks of human experience, which is to endow the external world, which is in and of itself profoundly alien to the self, with meaning. Throughout the course of life, one needs to project the subjective meaning of the inner self and the internal world into the whole "field" (1953, p. 91) of external reality. Without this projection, external reality is basically meaningless; experience of the "field," as barren and self-alien, would precipitate one's sense of loneliness and interrupt the flow of "being" and living.

For Winnicott, this "endowment of meaning" takes place through the projection of internal reality onto the external reality. The mechanisms of symbolization and representation allow for the experience of meaning and vitality in external reality; through these mechanisms, external reality will then act as a referent for something subjectively meaningful.

This then, is also the early developmental task of the infant; he must find a way to maintain the flow of "being" and project the vitality of internal reality in an external reality that he experiences in the context of separation from the mother and from a matrix of comfort and closeness. Again, for Winnicott, this is accomplished through the mechanisms of symbolism and representation, which help the infant endow objects (located in the external field) with subjective meaning. These objects then become cathected with meaning; they take on the character of being extensions of the self, its projections into the external "field." As such, they are "transitional," reflecting the character of the self moving into the world, of being both internal and external. Winnicott suggests that as the infant develops, and as the "field" between the child's internal and external reality continues to acquire greater subjective meaning, the initial transitional object itself becomes gradually "decathected" (1953, p. 97) and meaningless, since it is no longer the primary projection of internal psychical reality into the external world.

Importantly, Winnicott maintains that "transitional phenomena" (1953, p. 97), in the sense that there is an "intermediate" (1953, p. 89) area in between internal and external reality, play an important role in adult life as well. For example, Winnicott argues that the modes of experience present in artistic expression and creative work are connected to the child's capacity to endow the field of external reality with meaning and vitality, and to create a continuity between internal and external worlds.[5]

Winnicott theorizes that the capacity to experience and create transitional phenomena has its roots in the beginning stages of infancy, where the "good-enough mother" (1953, p. 94), through assiduous attention to and fulfillment of the infant's needs, allows the infant the "illusion" (1953, p. 94) of omnipotent control over her. Thus the infant experiences the mother as an object of the external world that, by responding to the infant's wishes and desires, is also a projection of his internal psychical reality.

Winnicott, in the context of Klein's discussion of the process of weaning, suggests that weaning provides the template for the mother's initiation of the gradual process of "disillusionment" (1953, p. 94). Ideally, the "good-enough mother" calibrates her withdrawal from the infant in such a way that it never experiences, in a sustained way, the frustrations of external reality as completely overwhelming and terrifying. As such, the process of weaning, and of the mother's gradual and calibrated withdrawal, helps mark the distinction between internal and external worlds (and in the process becomes a "not-me" relative to the infant), while allowing the child to maintain the sense that the external world can still fundamentally accommodate and absorb the projection and imposition of internal reality. He is then prepared for a healthy relationship with external reality.

Having laid out Winnicott's topography of inner and outer worlds, as well as the transitional world in between them, we can now introduce Winnicott's concept of the "false self." Winnicott (1965) suggests that the subjective experience of the self can be experienced in roughly two different ways. Ideally, subjective inner experience should be permeated by and allow sufficient access to sustained vitality, spontaneity, and creativity; under these circumstances, the self can be truly thought of as "alive." And yet, patients may report that they never felt alive, and that somehow their thoughts and feelings are not truly their own.

Winnicott relates these two modes of experience to two different psychical structures through which the self comes to be organized. These are the "True Self" and the "False Self," respectively. The True Self derives from "aliveness" (1965, p. 149) of the body and its responses to the sensorimotor stimuli experienced by the infant, as well the spontaneity and vitality of primary process thinking and intensity of id-driven desire. For Winnicott, the True Self can only meaningfully arise when mothering has been "good-enough," and has afforded the child early opportunities for the experience of "illusion," as we have outlined previously. Through this process the child lays down the groundwork for the meaningful engagement of inner psychical reality within external reality.

However, when the mother does not provide for the illusion of omnipotence, the consequence for the infant is a gradual alienation from the drives, fantasies, and needs of the inner (in the sense of "truer," or authentic) self. This occurs because the mother, under these circumstances, is demanding that the infant renounce his own needs and seek to gratify her own. What results then is that the infant (and eventually the adult) disengages from its own needs and internal reality, and instead learns to identify with and comply only (or primarily) with the mother's demands and needs. This alienation of the self from the vitality of its own inner reality, through exclusive (or primary) engagement with the demands of the social world leads to the feelings of deadness and hollowness that are engendered by the False Self. Winnicott explains that while to some degree, the False Self orientation is necessary to scaffold a successful compromise with the demands of reality, it becomes a pathological phenomenon when it no longer leaves room for the experience of the True Self.

Winnicott (as cited by Gergely & Watson, 1996) suggests that the mechanism for early experience of the True Self is the mirroring function that the mother provides for the infant. He suggests that ideally, a mother is able to mirror the child's affective experience in her facial expressions and bodily reactions, such that the child can then internalize a recognition of the self when it looks at the mother. This facilitates the "illusion of omnipotence" (1965, p. 146) by concretizing internal reality in external reality.

However, when the mother does not mirror the child's affect, the child is essentially flooded by the mother's affective experience, and his internal world is overwhelmed by the mother's projection of her own. As a consequence, the infant develops a sense of hopelessness at the futility of attempting to maintain a meaningful engagement with his own needs and wishes against the contingencies of external reality. Additionally, when there is insufficient maternal mirroring, the child is essentially internalizing and introjecting representations of the mother's emotional states, rather than his own. The consequence of these "non-self" internalizations, as highlighted by Bateman and Fonagy's (2006) description, is the presence within the ego of an "alien self," which produces a "sense of having feelings and ideas that . . . do not feel like one's own" (p. 15).

Gergely and Watson (1996), working within the framework of mentalization, further refine and expand Winnicott's suggestion of the importance of early maternal mirroring. They argue that the mechanism of maternal mirroring is critical for how children begin to recognize their own cognitive-affective states. They suggest that instinctively, mothers "mark" their mirroring of a child's state by reflecting it with a slight degree of exaggeration, either in facial expression or tone of voice. As such, the child learns to distinguish between the mother's own affective states (which are not exaggerated, but rather are "real") and this alternative pattern of reflection. Once this happens, the child is able to associate these "marked" reactions with their own actions, because of the contingent nature of the associative learning (the child's affective expressions repeatedly trigger the marked maternal reaction, and the marked maternal reaction is not triggered by anything else). As a consequence, the child can then gradually internalize representations of cognitive-affective states by linking their own internal states with the reflected states of the mother.

While the primary focus of Winnicott's analysis is on the "preoedipal" stage of development, and particularly the child's infant experiences of the mother, it would seem that the essential paradigm for falseness and alienation (as well as vitality and aliveness) suggested by Winnicott need not be restricted to the particular contours of those early stages. That is to say, for Winnicott, "being alive" has a specific meaning, and "being false" has a specific meaning. The sense of "aliveness" emerges from the presence of reliable pathways from internal to external; from impulse to action, from fantasy to play, and from the freedom to express affect and thought. Conversely, we might suggest that the constant suppression of impulse, shutting down of fantasy, and stifling of expression produce a "deadness" and an alienation, even if we shy away from describing a given person as profoundly "false." In other words, we are suggesting that compliance (as the proximal cause for self-censorship; either with internal or external demands) can produce a phenomenological state of deadness and alienation, even in instances where it does not produce a pervasive hollowness at the level of personality organization.[6]

This suggestion will allow us to consider the implications of his analysis for forms of psychopathology whose etiological pathways include later stages of development (and perhaps emerge later in development as well), and involve a lesser degree of personality pathology. More specifically, it will allow us to use Winnicott's thinking to help elucidate several aspects of the clinical phenomenology of OCD which we have noted to this point.

Similarly, Winnicott's analysis about the nature of meaning, while again rooted in the infant's relationship with the mother, can also be situated within the challenges of later phases in development. Indeed, Winnicott is explicit about the presence of and need for transitional phenomena within adult life. Accordingly, we can say that for Winnicott, the ability to invest the external world with subjective meaning, through the process of projecting the self into the field of external reality, is critical at all stages of human life.

Accordingly, in bringing to bear Winnicott's analysis to our discussion of OCD, we focus again on two aspects of OCD phenomenology: doubting (the primary object of our discussion) and compulsions (as the broader phenomenology of OCD symptomatology). We begin first by considering our discussion of doubting and uncertainty within the context of Winnicott's thought. We have suggested that a Kantian account of judgment best captures some of the central elements of OCD doubting and indecisiveness, including the kinds of judgments in which the struggle is with the problematical subsumption of a particular (often a circumstance or quality) under a known but [elusive] universal; with particular kinds of reflective judgments which, in the words of Beiner that we cited above, require one "to rise above particulars as given in sensory perception" (Beiner, 1983, p. 49).

In essence, then, we can suggest a transposition of Beiner's formulation into Winnicott's framework; that the "rising above particulars in sensory perception" requires a projection of the (subjective) internal world onto the external world. That is to say, the process of judgment involves moving from a place of (relative) objectivity, rooted in what is manifestly present and beyond debate, to a place of subjectivity. It requires the addition or input of internal, subjective mental content, which derives from internal processes of thought and feeling. And yet, making these sorts of reflective judgments requires one not merely to venture forth a purely subjective expression of agreeableness, but a determination which is to be intersubjectively valid, with the expectation that others *must* agree (despite the inherent inability to demonstrate the judgment's ultimate truth and validity). As such, difficulties with making these sorts of reflective judgments can be seen (from within Winnicott's framework) as a more fundamental difficulty with projecting the world of the self into the external world.

Moreover, we can connect our earlier discussion about how it comes to be that the child gains the confidence and trust in his own judgments to Winnicott's framework. We suggested that there emerges for the child (likely through the implicit and explicit feedback he receives from the parent) a sense that his own thinking begins to converge with that of his parents, that he has begun to reliably see the world as they do. At that point, he can begin to "cut out the middleman," so to speak, because he feels competent to reliably anticipate what his parents would say and how they would think. However, the absence of this convergence (experienced subjectively by the child), and the continued suspension of his judgment and deferral to that of the parent, would seem to create for the child a sense that his own reconstruction of reality is tentative and unreliable; it perpetuates a disjunction between internal and external worlds. In a sense then, we can suggest that the child's projection of his internal world (in the sense of how he subjectively reconstructs the external reality) into the external field is never really permitted to "land"; the continued pattern of suspending judgment and deferring to the parent perpetuates a lack of continuity between the child's inner world and his experience of the external world.

We now turn to a consideration of the implications of Winnicott's framework for the broader phenomenology of OCD symptomology, including the nature of compulsions. In the previous sections of this book, we have outlined some steps within a proposed developmental process in which the child "takes over" the parental "guiding" function. As part of the child's object-relation with the parent, the child recognizes in the parent, and endows the parent, with a certain authority; this authority is associated with the presence, in the parent (that is to say, in the child's representation of the parent), of certain qualities upon which this authority is constituted. These qualities include the parent's knowledge of things, their competence, and so on. We have suggested the child's taking over of these functions is linked to a sense which develops for the child, that he is sufficiently "like" the parent such that his actions and determinations will lead to the same positive outcomes associated with the parent; that the child comes to feel that he has a sufficient degree of "competence," approximating that of the parent, to guide his own behavior and make his own judgments.

There are two steps of this process which are particularly connected to the themes we have outlined here in our presentation of Winnicott. These are the child's capacity to restrain his own impulses and subordinate his own "sense of things" in deference to the parent's authority, and the a priori legitimacy accorded to the parent's directives and judgments, which is eventually afforded to oneself when the process of internalization has been completed.

As we have suggested, part of the child's acceptance of the adult's authority is the emergence of the child's capacity to internally align themselves with the expectations and demands of the adult, over and against their own impulses. Ideally, the emergence of this capacity leads to changes in the child's motivational structure, as described by Schafer, and the crystallization of the child's conscience as a central structural component of the self. However, this process might also come, at times, at significant cost; it is possible that the child becomes too adept at the stifling of his own impulses, and can become significantly alienated from his own capacity for spontaneity. The "motivating sphere of consciousness" (Vygotsky, p. 107) itself may begin to feel self-alien, perhaps even threatening. Synthesizing earlier elements of our account, we can readily conjure a picture in which every motive, thought, and impulse needs to be checked against the demands and injunctions of a looming presence of an introjected parental authority within the boundaries of the self-as-place.[7] In a sense, the effect is similar to the "flooding" the infant might experience in the dyadic relationship with a demanding and controlling mother whose presence overwhelms the child's own inner world, and generates the emergence of the False Self.

We can conjure as well how this sense of alienation from one's own animating impulses and capacity for spontaneity can give rise to an inner life that is marked by an exaggerated adherence to rules and avoidance of spontaneity; in essence, then, a form of excessive rigidity. We provide here Shapiro's characterization of this form of obsessional rigidity:

> In ritual and only less acutely in ordinary compulsive purposefulness, the individual feels, in contrast to normal experience, like a servant of his purpose. He feels the responsibility that the dutiful soldier feels to satisfy military regulations, quite apart from whether he knows their reasons . . . . But in neither of these cases is there a sense of genuine self-direction or choice, except as the executor of assigned responsibility. The sense of duty, or of responsibility to superior authority, in this sense, dilutes the experience of personal choice and motivation, or supplants it in consciousness altogether, even while it intensifies the experience of failure. (p. 78)

Shapiro describes further the particular contours of a consciousness permeated by "should's and should not's":

> It is a conscientiousness of rules, something quite different from a conscientiousness of personal conviction. A conscientiousness of rules dilutes or displaces the normal experiences of personal choice and agency, whereas the ordinary conscience participates in that experience. (p. 79)

As Shapiro explains, this exaggerated "conscientiousness of rules" leads to an experience of the world in which there is a disembodied quality to rules; for the compulsive, they are not fully contextualized or rooted in purpose and goals. That being said, it is important to clarify as well within the context of

Shapiro's description that experiencing a sense of duty to a higher purpose (as well as religious devotion) is qualitatively different than the form of consciousness which we are discussing here; that is, a way of being and thinking which is structured around the inhibition of spontaneity and creativity, and does not even allow for the sense of meaning and fulfilment which comes from the sense of duty and the identification with a higher purpose.

As Shapiro explains further, instead of becoming aware of the rule as it is occasioned organically in the natural course of events, there is an a priori maintenance of rule-awareness which occupies a significant degree of mental space:

> It requires a continual awareness of the existence of those rules, a continual awareness of should's. This is evident in the obsessive-compulsive person's continual reminding of himself, nagging of himself, that he "should" do this or that. His consciousness of rules has the effect of transforming them into demanding imperatives ("You should do!"). (p. 80)

Here, Shapiro is charting a pathway from the crystallization of a rule-bound consciousness to the experience of compulsions. We may outline it as follows: we can think of a person (a child or an adult) who maintains in their mind an awareness of cleanliness and hygiene-related rules. For instance, coming into contact with dirt is unclean and unsafe, and requires cleansing. Given the seriousness of the risk of germs, this particular rule has a high degree of salience for him; as such, he is frequently on the lookout for possible instances of "becoming dirty." Rather than invoking this rule when he feels himself to have become dirty, he has reversed the process, and is always wondering whether he has become dirty, and whether the "rule" needs to be applied.

Moreover, the actual initiation of the cleansing process, under these conditions, reflects a particular quality of motivation. It is something that he feels "compelled" to do, in the sense of doing it for an external reason, to satisfy an external demand, as the initiation of the behavior program (e.g., hand-washing) does not arise organically from within the natural course of events. Accordingly, the task's completion is not measured in reference to his own immediate goals and motivations. Rather, it is measured in reference to some quasi-objective standard, determined by some external person or principle; for example, "how clean must one's hands be," or that there is an objective standard of ascertainable cleanliness which successful hand-washing must meet. As such, there can never be any real completion of the hand-washing task; the person's loss of motivation (for whatever reason), which normally ends the task (maybe he feels clean, or is in a rush, or stops being worried, or has run out of water or soap), is irrelevant in compulsive washing, since the action itself never emerged from his own internal motivation, but was always a "soldier-like" performance of duty. The compulsive washer is thus impervious to the organic environmental cues which generally provide the feedback necessary to end a given task.

Moreover, we can suggest as well another point about the nature of compulsive motivation. That is to say, embedded within the qualitative structure of compulsive motivations is that as a motivational system (of an aggregation of individual motives), they do not in them themselves constitute a concrete set of goals which stimulate and guide behavior. Rather, they reflect desires for the attainment of states in which no further action needs to be taken. For instance, the desire to be clean, or safe, or innocent of a potential misdeed, are in essence desires for the *absence* of something, rather the presence of something; for example, the absence of germs, the cessation of threatening fears, the absence of aggression, or the removal of a potential punishment. In other words, these desires really reflect a more fundamental desire to "get rid" of something, to "finally finish" with something, to discharge some burden or weight. This, too, can be seen as an expression of the compulsive's diminished volition and sense of agency. He is not looking to bend the world to suit his needs (or to better the world around him), but to free himself from the impositions of the world.

This formulation can be connected to Winnicott's notion of the transitional field. We can say that the compulsive does not see external reality as inviting or receptive to the projections of his internal world, and therefore does not experience himself as an active participant in it. Rather, he is threatened by it; by its dirt, by its germs, by its demands, and so on. He does what he can to restore himself to states of selfhood that are pure and unsullied by involvement with external reality.

The particular qualities of this form of motivation also address the question we restated in our summary of Vygotsky about the nature of compulsions.[8] There is a subjective experience of a motivational structure that is devoted to the soldier-like fulfillment of demands and requirements that emanate from inside the mind (in the sense that rule-salience and rule-awareness are rigorously maintained; and it is the self which actually initiates the behavioral programs), but whose purpose and function does not emerge in responses to the impulses and desire which generally serve to motivate behavior. They are therefore experienced as arising independently of the self's own "motivating sphere."

Returning to Winnicott, we can begin to think about how a person finds himself in this state of being. Again, while it does not necessarily converge with Winnicott's description of the False Self, we will make use of our suggestion that Winnicott's description also provides a more general paradigm of alienation and diminished agency.

In essence, we are describing a sense of powerlessness and a subjective loss of agency.[9] Within the framework of the child's acceptance of the adult's authority, we can think of the child's relationship with the parent (in the sense of an object-relation) as drawing heavily (or significantly colored by) from the child's experiences of having been made to complete tasks which he felt to be idiosyncratic, whose completion was met with harsh evaluation, and seemingly (to the child) opaque determinations which the child felt unable to grasp. Demands were likely made with an intensity that conveyed the seriousness and gravity of the tasks, and the threat of stern disapproval for failing to carry them out. In these situations, the child likely experienced himself as having no choice but to comply. There was no possible way of saying "I'm not in the mood"; the demands thus constituted an intrusion into the child's inner world, flooding him in a manner parallel to that of a more generally intrusive parent (described by Winnicott). They likely overwhelmed the child's own motives and goals, as well as his own ability to determine the appropriate end of the task ("you're not done yet, you missed a spot here, and a spot there, and another one here"), and produced a sense of alienation from the "motivating sphere" of his own consciousness. While this framework (as well as the more impressionistic composite illustration of this particular pattern of formative experiences and interactions)[10] clearly cannot account for the full range of compulsions and OCD symptomatology, we can suggest that it explicates and amplifies some of the central experiences and dynamics of OCD presentations.

As we have mentioned, Winnicott's account also connects to the nature of the "a priori" legitimacy accorded to the authority of the parent, and ideally reacquired by the child themselves. That is to say, the fundamental attitude of confidence in one's knowledge, in the efficacy of their actions, and in the validity of their choices, seems to draw upon a basic sense of rootedness in the world; that impulses and desires can "land" in the external world, without being destroyed, or leading to his own destruction. In other words, the fundamental sense that there is a basic legitimacy and viability to the impulses that animate inner life, and that living safely in the external world does not require self-erasure.

Relatedly, we can suggest that the themes of OCD obsessions and compulsions, including the excessive preoccupations with safety or with one's moral state and the profound and pervasive experience of doubting and uncertainty (both about reality, as well as the efficacy of one's actions, "did I lock the door?") can be seen as reflective of a fundamental lack of rootedness in the world, and of a profound form of self-erasure. Moreover, compulsive doubting can be seen in this way as well, as we have suggested. The tentative nature of the self's projections of inner reality into the external field results in a disjunction between inner and outer worlds, which results in a persistent sense of instability surrounding the self's rendering of external reality. And lastly, in moral compulsions, such as wondering about having mistakenly driven over someone and hurt or killed them, there is an implicit idea that perhaps the world itself is better off without the compulsive's involvement (e.g., the very act of driving to work becomes problematic, and should be avoided so as not to cause harm). In compulsive checking, the pervasive sense of wondering whether a given action was performed correctly, or that it was effective, reflects a fundamental tentativeness in one's ability to shape the world, as we have suggested.

Importantly, while much of our discussion linking the implications of Winnicott's theory to the phenomenology of OCD has centered on the self's tentative projection into the world, Winnicott's thinking about the essential emergence of the self also has significant implications for our consideration of OCD symptoms. Specifically, we have outlined how for Winnicott the child's ego (as a structure) as well as their sense of reality as coherent and ordered emerges from the mother's organization of the child's somatic and sensory experiences through the building up of caretaking routines, and that achieving this "continuity of being" is one of the central tasks of the "holding phase." Accordingly, Winnicott's thinking suggests that we can also think about pervasive states of doubting and chronic uncertainty within the context of these early experiences as well. We can readily imagine how an anxious caregiver may themselves experience caretaking routines with a sense of worry and heightened concern, and how this anxiety may be transmitted to the infant. If the mother becomes overwhelmed and flooded by thoughts and worries related to her caring for the infant, her anxiety may permeate the "holding environment"; the infant's experience of mundane routine may become punctuated by the intermittent flashes of worry and concern he may perceive in the mother. Indeed, this particular pattern of mundane routine and suddenly precarious existence (the sense that something routine may become suddenly frightening), as well as the acute awareness of the stakes involved in the proper performance of the routine, call to mind several salient characteristics of OCD, including concerns about safety and health, as well as the role of ritual and routine.

Relatedly, we mentioned that for Winnicott, the infant's ability to maintain a sense of its own "continuity" in the process of separation from the mother is to a large degree dependent on its ability to hold on to the imago-representation of the mother. Furthermore, this ability is itself dependent on the reinforcement of the "actual mother" and her caretaking. That is to say, it is the mother's caretaking that bolsters the infant's ego and helps the infant maintain an integrated and coherent sense of reality while warding off states of psychical dissolution and disintegration. We can now suggest a link between the process of creating this integrated sense of reality, and the phenomenology of doubting. That is to say, states of pervasive and intense doubting may lead to a sense of disintegration and dissolution, as the ordered rendering of reality begins to collapse.

As such, we can make two points here. The first is in connection to the "a priori" legitimacy accorded to the parent, which we have outlined earlier. Winnicott's identification of the mother's role in maintaining the infant's "continuity of being" suggests another point in development in which the child "outsources" the rendering of reality to the parent, as it relies on the parent to create a world of order and clarity while staving off disintegration. Secondly, it suggests that the ability to create an ordered and clear reality, one marked by well-defined expectations and meanings, is an achievement of the infant's developing ego, scaffolded by the maternal ego. Accordingly, successfully attaining and holding on to states of certainty can be related to the consolidation of ego strength in this period of the "holding phase." Conversely, difficulty with maintaining these states of certainty and "knowing" may be seen as emerging from suboptimal consolidation of this aspect of ego functioning.[11]

NOTES

1. For this discussion, we draw primarily from Winnicott's (1960) paper, The Theory of the Parent-Infant Relationship.

2. Though the paper itself was published in 1960, we cite here the paper as it appears in the collection The Maturational Processes and the Facilitating Environment, published in 1965.

3. In his 1960 paper, Winnicott describes the *internalized* "build-up in the infant of memories of maternal care," "accumulation of memories of care," and "introjection of care details" (p. 590) as critically facilitative of the infant's independent self. Of note in relation to our discussion at the conclusion of the chapter, Winnicott includes the following term in his description of the outcome of this process of internalization: "the development of confidence in the environment" (p. 590).

4. We will describe this process more fully in our discussion of transitional phenomena.

5. Interestingly, Winnicott does draw a connection between transitional phenomena and OCD rituals (see p. 91). However, he does not elaborate, and seems to refer to the quality of reassurance provided by the ritual rather than the direction we have suggested here.

6. Indeed, Winnicott himself is clear that the issue of "falseness" is one of degree and is not binary. He suggests that in the normal course of development, the processes of socialization require the child to develop the capacity for a degree of compliance with external demands. Relatedly, Winnicott maintains that "falseness" can have serious consequences for personality even if it does not completely obscure the "true self." For instance, he suggests that for some actors, notwithstanding the sense of

vitality to which they have access while performing, there is a nonetheless a pervasive sense of emptiness in their daily lives.

7. Indeed, as we have suggested in our earlier discussion of Schafer, and as we will revisit in the last chapter, the potential presence of a commanding, judging, and intrusive parental introject readily maps onto the phenomenology of OCD compulsions. This also relates to the next point made in our discussion of motivation, since the motivation animating the compulsion might be "assigned" to the introject, and not to the self-as-agent.

8. This pathway is less clear in idiosyncratic compulsions, such as counting rituals.

9. As described by Shapiro, referenced above.

10. Of note, see Basile et al. (2017, citing Tenore, 2016) who state: "It is quite common that OCD patients report early negative experiences with their caregivers have been particularly punitive and critical..." (p. 412).

11. We note here within the context of Winnicott's notion of "good enough" parenting (see above, p. 136) that generally speaking one would expect children to achieve sufficient ego consolidation at this stage. It is only with regard to clinically significant difficulties with doubting and OCD symptoms to which we suggest a link to suboptimal consolidation of ego strength at this stage of development.

Chapter 6

In Conclusion

Implications for Treatment

At this point in our discussion, we can now begin to trace some implications for treatment which emerge from our account. Given that our account draws heavily from psychodynamic theory, we begin first with a brief overview of the broad psychodynamic approach to the treatment of OCD. As we have mentioned in the opening section of this book, the psychodynamic approach to OCD has generally emphasized the critical effect of intrapsychic conflict in the etiology and structure of OCD symptomatology. King, in his overview (2017) of psychodynamic approaches to OCD, provides the following summary:

> The psychodynamic perspective on obsessive-compulsive disorder (OCD) seeks to understand OC phenomena in terms of conflicting intrapsychic motives or personal imperatives, with an emphasis on characteristic coping or defensive styles and the developmental vicissitudes of conscience and culture.

These conflicts revolve around thoughts or wishes which are experienced as threatening to the self, and which may provoke intense anxiety, guilt, or shame. These often consist of aggressive or ambivalent feelings toward loved ones, thoughts of rebellion, or sexual content. Accordingly, the manifestation of these thoughts activates the ego's defenses, as it attempts to ward off and shut down the offending impulse or keep the thought out of awareness, and thereby reduce the tension which it may cause. As King further describes:

> If, in this struggle to ward off anxiety stirred by seemingly dangerous or transgressive impulses, the individual resorts heavily to specific characteristic coping or defense mechanisms—such as undoing, reaction formation, isolation of

111

affect/intellectualization, doubting, or magical thinking—obsessive-compulsive character traits or symptoms may result.

That is to say, the success of this "heavy" reliance on these mechanisms of defense is tenuous and fleeting, and results in distortions of character and personality, as well as the constellation of OCD symptoms.

Importantly, there is heterogeneity among psychodynamic theories regarding the specific patterns of aversive impulses and the corresponding defenses which are engaged. As King explains, citing Millon (2011):

> Different authors have emphasized different aspects of the conflict(s) and maladaptive response(s) hypothesized to underlie OC phenomena; hence there is no single, unified psychodynamic theory of OCD, or even consensus about what the obsessional patient fears and must guard against most.

Accordingly, a psychodynamic approach to treatment would concentrate on the nature of the conflict, rather than on managing the particular cluster of behavioral symptoms which have emerged. It will aim to move the conflict from the shadows to the open, and give the patient the insight to work through and resolve the conflict through other means, without the distortions created by obsessive defenses. This insight would help the patient recognize and understand the links between their obsessive or compulsive symptoms and the underlying conflicts from which they arise. For instance, if a patient experiences obsessions about whether they "had a thought" to hurt a loved one, a psychodynamic approach would aim to help the patient become aware of potential feelings of aggression toward the person he loves, as well as the particular pattern of defenses which are activated to keep these feelings out of awareness.

To clarify further, this does not imply that the patient should necessarily identify with the aggressive feelings. There are of course impulses, thoughts, or desires that may in fact be morally aversive and one's guilt in fact would be well-placed in response. In such an instance, a dynamic approach would likely focus on the distortions of mind and experience which take place as a byproduct of the patient's pattern of defense. Accordingly, we may hope for the patient to be able to work through their conflict in a more adaptive manner, such as through moral, rather than obsessive, struggle. Moreover, within OCD, as we have mentioned, the patient may not feel subjectively that there is any potential reality in carrying out the (even appropriately) proscribed wish or thought, but is disturbed by the presence and discovery of a feeling of aggression towards a loved one. In such an instance, it would be helpful for the patient to better understand the source of these aggressive feelings as well as he assumptions which prompt him to defend against them so intensely (such as a fear that that the relationship with the loved one is so fragile that it could not withstand any expression of aggression or survive any friction).

In this context, it bears mention that there has been a recent effort to introduce a shorter-term, more specific and targeted psychodynamic therapy for OCD. Leichsenring and Steinert (2017) have proposed a targeted, modular treatment which draws upon Luborsky's (1984) models of shorter-term psychodynamic therapy. Following Luborsky's (1984) methods for efficiently identifying and articulating CCRT's (core conflictual relational themes), they outline a treatment module which is centered around identifying and working through the core central conflicts which underlie a given patient's OCD presentation. According to Leichsenring and Steinert, these themes often revolve around either "a rigid superego" (p. 361) and threatening thoughts or impulses, as well as themes of control and autonomy.

As part of their treatment, Leichsenring and Steinert do also explicitly aim to incorporate elements of the object-relations involved in OCD. Specifically, they suggest (citing Lang, 2015) that exploring in an "accepting and non-condemning way"[2] (p. 365) the patient's expectations of responses (from both the therapist and others in their lives) to the disclosures of threatening feelings and thoughts will provide the opportunity both to improve reality testing as well as for "corrective emotional experiences" (p. 365), as invariably the responses they receive will be much gentler than those they expect. This in turn will help "mitigate the strictness" (p. 365) of superego functioning. Leichsenring and Steiner's point here seems particularly relevant to the often idiosyncratic or exaggerated fantasies of catastrophe expected by OCD patients in response to violating their compulsions. Relatedly, we note as well here that their discussion about "mitigating the strictness" of a "rigid superego" does not imply a laxity in adherence to ethical norms and principles, but rather relates to the particularly punitive and aggressive quality of the self-criticism experienced within OCD. That being said, their approach does not engage with the fuller account of object-relations which seems present in OCD, including the nature of identification with parental figures and the likely presence of introjects, in the sense used by Schafer.[3]

This point can be made more broadly about the general psychodynamic approach to OCD, as described by King (2017), that while psychodynamic theory has highlighted the role of intrapsychic *conflict* within the symptomatology of OCD, and provides the tools to make sense of the meaning and symbolism of specific OCD obsessions and compulsions, it seems to have given considerably less attention to the intrapsychic *structure* present in OCD. As we have suggested, the processes of internalization, including those of identification and introjection, seem to be central to a more thorough understanding of the specific qualitative structure of the superego within OCD, as well as the particular nature in which self and other are experienced within the phenomenologies of doubting and compulsion.

As such, we are not suggesting that the structural characteristics and representations of self and other which we have proposed should supplant or obviate the conflict-based approach to OCD that has been at the center of psychodynamic approaches since Freud. Similarly, it is also not the intention of this work to suggest an account that by itself is sufficient to explain all aspects of the disorder. Rather, we are suggesting that these phenomena are real and meaningful, and that they constitute an important aspect of the clinical picture which has not received as much theoretical attention as perhaps it should have received. In essence, the account we present is fundamentally psychodynamic, and should be seen as an attempt to use existing theory to more fully explicate aspects of symptomatology, rather than as an attempt to introduce a new metapsychology.

Accordingly, within the context of a treatment approach, we are suggesting that the focus of a psychodynamic treatment of OCD be widened. While still exploring the central conflicts that may be at the core of any given clinical presentation, we suggest (on the basis of our account) that attention should also be paid to the specific structural characteristics and representations of self and other (including superego structure and the nature of identifications and possible introjects) which may surface as well.

By way of illustration, the incorporation of a mentalization-based approach (following the general principles outlined by Bateman & Fonagy, 2006) intended to scaffold the emergence of a patient's "observing ego" and encourage the patient's curiosity about the workings of their own mind, would provide a way for patients to begin to engage with the boundaries of self and other within the topographies of their own minds. Potentially, this curiosity would help patients better clarify the nature of a compulsion. Here are a few questions which might be explored more explicitly in work with OCD patients:

Is the compulsion coming from inside, or from outside? And if it is from outside, how did it "get in"? Has it always been "inside"? Do the demands or the doubting sometimes get worse? If so, when? And why?

Having the patient explore these questions in the course of a treatment should help create some meaningful space away from the suffocating presence of the "commanding" figure or voice which expresses the compulsive demands, and move past the concreteness and "reality" of their presence.

Additionally, a mentalization-based approach provides a framework for exploring the patient's idiosyncratic rendering of the consequences of disobeying compulsion. Exploring questions such as "What happens if you say no, what will happen? How do you know that this will happen?" and so on, with an attitude not of skepticism or incredulity (which might lead to shame and resistance) but with genuine curiosity and openness provides a way for patients to begin to ask these questions themselves. While this overlaps to some degree with the approach suggested by Leichsenring and Steiner, this framework provides an additional pathway through which to address the particular qualities of the OCD superego. The intention here is for the patient, through the development of their observing ego, to dull the intensity of the compulsive commands, and move away from the immediacy and palpability of the anticipated catastrophe. Essentially, we are suggesting a process through which the patient will move from the pressured and harrowing experience of compulsions, to creating and learning to inhabit a more contemplative mental space.

There are two additional advantages to the incorporation of this approach. The first is that within OCD, it is common for patients to present with poor insight (Leichsenring & Steinert, 2007, citing Stein, 2002), which often stands in the way of treatment. A mentalization-based approach which aims to help the patient gradually learn the nature of their own mind would provide a means of improving insight. In this sense, such an approach could even be used adjunctively with a CBT or behaviorally-oriented treatment. Of note, some cognitive-behavioral models of treatment, including one suggested by Wagner (2003, citing Schwartz, 1996), also emphasize the importance of "renaming" OCD thoughts and "externalizing" (Wagner, 2003, p. 295) them (by assigning them to the "worry monster" or to "OCD" rather than the "rational self") with the similar goal of enhancing insight and awareness of their irrationality.[4] Secondly, a gentle, more exploratory approach to the consequences of disregarding a compulsion would offer a more collaborative and less threatening environment for "imaginal exposure,"[5] response prevention, and extinction than a more directive behavioral treatment.

Furthermore, treatment should also explore the qualities of the commanding figure or voice (or any other representation), if these are the means through which the compulsion is expressed. In the course of our discussion we have suggested that various representations of others, located within the self-as-place, often express the compulsive command. We have argued that the ways in which parts of the mind can be experienced as self-alien within OCD symptomatology seem critical for a fuller picture of the nature of intrusive thoughts which form the core of OCD obsessions. We provide here the following illustration of the self-alien nature of intrusive thoughts, drawn from a first-person account of OCD struggles and recovery. Given that the "personalization" of OCD is conceptually tangential to the models and mechanisms of the exposure and response prevention framework for OCD, patient descriptions of "personified" OCD elements are not typically presented in articles or case vignettes. Additionally, while descriptions of OCD compulsions (see Shapiro, 2000) readily articulate the perceived loss of agency and sense of "feeling forced" to perform rituals, there is less attention paid to "who" or "what" is doing the "compelling." As such, we present portions of an account which gives voice to the "personified" elements of OCD. This account, authored by Kirsten Pagacz (2016), exhaustively details her

OCD symptoms, and narrates their trajectory through her treatment (CBT and exposure therapy) and recovery. The "personification" of her OCD symptoms is central to her account, as well as to her recovery, as we will see.

The author describes the experience and presence of an almost-autonomous object, whom she refers to as "Sergeant,"[6] and who directs her OCD behavior, which gives expression to the sense of a self-alien presence, seemingly located in the liminal space between self and other:

> Sergeant commanded my attention and controlled the switch at my reward and punishment center in what seemed to be the deepest part of my brain. This was our relationship and it had been like this for more than ten years and going strong. . . . I would just follow his commands and orders. It was just easier this way. Otherwise, he would force-feed me obsessive thought after obsessive thought and my head would truly overload and it was not unlikely for me to break down crying. (p. 55)

Later in her narrative, the author describes a conversation she had as a young adult, while suffering intensely from her OCD symptoms, in which she refers to a "wild monkey presence inside me":

> What was bothering me so? We would shine a light inside the dark tunnel of my being, and he (*what felt like a wild monkey*) would jump to the next corner. Something was there, something was wild, and it was something we had never seen before, something that had control, and something that was leading my life. I caught glimpses of his wild hair, but that was all . . . . As we talked about this wild monkey presence inside me, I tried to describe how he would completely take over my thinking, even my breath at times. (pp 69–70)

These descriptions center on themes of reward and punishment, commanding and complying. From within our framework, these descriptions are suggestive of the presence of a superego that has been personified and is experienced as an object with whom these themes are played out. In other words, it would seem that according to Schafer, what is being described is the likely continuation or reenactment of themes in relationships with others, as they are reconstituted and played out internally, with an object-representation. Moreover, this object-representation is described as external to the self-as-agent but internal to the self-as-place; the author has a sense that "Sergeant" is permanently inside of her, and that she cannot escape or evade him. Thus, we can say that for Schafer, "Sergeant" seems to have the structural characteristics of a "presence," and is likely a harsh introject.

Importantly, the author suggests that acknowledging the self-alien characteristics of OCD, at the suggestion of her therapist, helped play a role in her recovery:[7]

giving a name to your tormentor may help you to separate from it/him/her. My OCD is called Monkey. That's the name I thought described him best. This separation, of giving him a name, brought some awareness and relief to the forefront. (pp. 98–99)

We suggest therefore that the treatment explore more fully the particular patterns of interaction between the patient and important figures from the patient's childhood from which this introject, or presence, is likely derived. An approach derived from Kernberg's (2015) TFP would have as its goal bringing about the integration, dissolution, or accommodation (in which the figure assumes a more benign, less malicious and threatening presence) of the commanding presence, should one be present.

Interestingly, over the past several years, there has been an emerging literature on the treatment of OCD with Schema Therapy approaches, which aims to address the range of patients who do not respond to more behaviorally oriented treatments, as well those with comorbid personality disorders (Basile et al., 2017). Schema Therapy, or ST, has been defined as "a third wave CBT approach that combines different models, that is, gestalt and attachment theories, emotion-focused, cognitive and behavioral strategies" (Basile et al., 2017, p. 407). It focuses on Early Maladaptive Schemas (EMS) of internalized parental modes, associated feelings, and learned responses and coping mechanisms. Among these are the critical/punitive parent mode, which "refers to the parental introjected rules on being punished for possible mistakes" (Basile et al., p. 412), and the demanding parent mode, which "reflects the internalized parental voices related to pressure to achieve unrealistically high expectations" (Basile et al., 2017, p. 412; see as well our discussion in note 1, where we clarified that the emphasis here is on the function of rules specifically within OCD, which is to maintain a sense of control and avoid vulnerability). Basile et al. (2017), following Gross et al. (2012) theorize that in OCD, the experience of these parental modes in turn activate specific "child modes," including a vulnerable child mode, a perfectionistic/overcontroller mode, and an angry/detached protector mode. According to Basile et al. (2017), it is these child modes which account for OCD symptomatology. For instance, they describe here the theorized pathway from the perfectionistic mode to OCD symptoms:

The over-compensatory coping mode is designed to create as much distance as possible from feelings of vulnerability, through cultivating a sense of being "in control." This process takes place through perfectionism, rituals, rumination, superstitious thinking, and focusing on rules and regulations at the expense of health, happiness, and human connection. (p. 412, see note 2, above)

Gross et al. (2012) provide a case illustration of their model:

Mary B. is a thirty-one-year-old, currently unemployed bank assistant. She has suffered severe compulsions and coexisting obsessions for twenty years. She washes her hands up to forty times a day, combining it with a counting ritual. Her washing and cleaning relate particularly to a fear of contamination with different pathogens or poisonous substances. She is also obsessed with checking and controlling. Her OCD leaves her socially isolated. She suffers from depressive symptoms (e.g., suicidal thoughts) as well as aggressive impulses, which lead to self-harming behavior (cutting or burning herself) to regulate emotional stress in harmful interpersonal relationships. Her father died from cancer when Mary was eleven years old. She felt guilty and responsible for his death, because she remembered having touched his knee the day before he died. After his death, she developed the compulsions and began isolating herself. (p. 176)

Among their interpretations of Mary's symptoms, Gross et al. (2012) suggest the following schema-based approach:

In talking about functionality it was shown that Mary needs the OCD to calm her Demanding Parent mode that urges her to achieve certain unrelenting standards. This mode resembles her mother's voice from when Mary was young. Mary always had to fulfill her mother's wishes, not daring to stand up for herself. Her OCD "helps" her to reject requirements and to regulate distance to others, and therefore creates a sense of apparent control and autonomy. (p. 176)

Returning to our discussion, we might suggest that these two related parental modes theorized by Basile et al. (2017, following Gross et al., 2012), who describes them as "introjected," emerge from the processes of internalization which we have outlined in Schafer. In this context, the suggestion that Mary's voice "resembles" her mother's critical voice takes on particular salience. Furthermore, following Schafer, we argue that it is insufficient merely to describe these modes as "schematic"; rather, especially within the context of OCD, attention must be paid to the concrete (though subjective) reality of these non-self-representations in the mind. Specifically, the way in which the internalized parental figures mediate (and obstruct) the normal functioning of motivational and cognitive elements of mind, including the ability to render judgments and make determinations, must be taken into account for a phenomenologically and conceptually richer rendering of OCD symptomatology. By placing much of OCD symptomatology within the realm of the processes of internalization, introjection, and identification, we believe we are rendering to the disorder a much-warranted object relational component. This component, in turn, can help highlight the continuities between the often confounding and peculiar behaviors of OCD and the more familiar phenomena of doubt and indecision embedded within human experience. Seen through this lens, OCD then becomes less opaque and less alienating, to others and to the sufferer. The more fully we can render the phenomenological experience of OCD, the more humanely we can then treat it.

NOTES

1. More broadly, see again our comments on p. 112–113 regarding morally aversive thoughts and desires, as well as Huppert et al. (2007) for a discussion about OCD and aversive thoughts within a religious context. Similarly, with regard to the suggestion made by Basile et al. (2017) about "focusing on rules and regulations" (referenced in our discussion below, p. 117), we note that the development of rule-bound behavior and thought is an important and necessary achievement (and way of being), and that the discussion here concerns the excessive and clinically significant distortions within OCD.

2. Though a broader analysis of this specific treatment approach is beyond the scope of our discussion, we have cited the study to contextualize our focus on the object-relational elements of the OCD superego.

3. We are suggesting though that this externalizing effects structural change, rather than merely cognitive change. Nonetheless, one advantage of this approach is that it does overlap in "how it looks" with elements of CBT treatments.

4. See Hupert et al. (2007) for an explanation of this concept. Briefly, it refers to exposures done when "in vivo" exposures are not possible.

5. Importantly it seems as if the name "Sergeant" was assigned to this presence only in the process of writing the book (p. 69). Nonetheless, it seems clear from her account, especially her discussion of "Stranger"(p. 3), the "monkey presence"(p. 69), as well as her descriptions of the sense of company and amelioration of loneliness (p. 144) provided by this presence and the sense of "mourning" in response to its absence, that she is describing an object/presence as much as a metaphor. That is to say, that the author's descriptions would not be substantively meaningful if used to describe other disorders, such as depression. See as well her comments that "telling on it is wrong" (p. 100). Accordingly, it would seem that Schafer would categorize this experience as that of a presence or an introject.

6. The author seems to be describing the suggestion she received in the course of her own therapy, and seems to be the same technique referenced above in our discussion of Wagner (2003), citing Schwartz (1996).

References

Aardema, F., & O'Connor, K. (2012). Dissolving the tenacity of obsessional doubt: Implications for treatment outcome. *Journal of Behavior Therapy and Experimental Psychiatry, 43*(2), 855–861.

Abramovitch, A., Abramowitz, J. S., & Mittelman, A. (2013). The neuropsychology of adult obsessive–compulsive disorder: A meta-analysis. *Clinical Psychology Review, 33*(8), 1163–1171.

Abramovitch, A., & Cooperman, A. (2015). The cognitive neuropsychology of obsessive-compulsive disorder: A critical review. *Journal of Obsessive-Compulsive and Related Disorders, 5*, 24–36.

Abramowitz, J. S., Taylor, S., & McKay, D. (2009). Obsessive-compulsive disorder. *Lancet, 374*(9), 491–499.

Allison, H. E. (2001). *Kant's theory of taste: A reading of the Critique of aesthetic judgment.* Cambridge University Press.

American Psychiatric Association. (2013). *Diagnostic and statistical manual of mental disorders* (5th ed.). American Psychiatric Association.

Basile, B., Tenore, K., Luppino, O. I., & Mancini, F. (2017). Schema therapy mode model applied to OCD. *Clinical Neuropsychiatry, 14*(6), 407–414.

Bateman, A., & Fonagy, P. (2010). Mentalization based treatment for borderline personality disorder. *World Psychiatry, 5*, 11–15.

Beiner, R. (1983). *Political judgment.* The University of Chicago Press.

Berk, L. E., & Garvin, R. A. (1994). Development of private speech among low-income Appalachian children. *Developmental Psychology, 20*(2), 271–286.

Buhr, K., & Dugas, M. J. (2009). The role of fear of anxiety and intolerance of uncertainty in worry: An experimental manipulation. *Behaviour Research and Therapy, 47*(3), 215–223.

Chamberlain, S. R., Blackwell, A. D., Fineberg, N. A., Robbins, T. W., & Sahakian, B. J. (2005). The neuropsychology of obsessive compulsive disorder: The importance of failures in cognitive and behavioural inhibition as candidate endophenotypic markers. *Neuroscience & Biobehavioral Reviews, 29*(3), 399–419.

Coles, M. E., Frost, R. O., Heimberg, R. G., & Rhéaume, J. (2003). "Not just right experiences": Perfectionism, obsessive–compulsive features and general psychopathology. *Behaviour Research and Therapy, 41*(6), 681–700.

Dar, R., Rish, S., Hermesh, H., Taub, M., & Fux, M. (2000). Realism of confidence in obsessive-compulsive checkers. *Journal of Abnormal Psychology, 109*(4), 673–678.

Doron, G., Derby, D. S., & Szepsenwol, O. (2014). Relationship obsessive compulsive disorder (ROCD): A conceptual framework. *Journal of Obsessive-Compulsive and Related Disorders, 3*(2), 169–180.

Edwards, A. (2007). An interesting resemblance: Vygotsky, Mead, and American pragmatism. In H. Daniels, M. Cole, & J. V. Wertsch (Eds.), *The Cambridge companion to Vygotsky* (1st ed., pp. 77–100). Cambridge University Press.

Exner, C., Martin, V., & Rief, W. (2009). Self-focused ruminations and memory deficits in obsessive–compulsive disorder. *Cognitive Therapy and Research, 33*(2), 163–174.

Freud, S. (1909). Notes upon a case of obsessional neurosis. In J. Strachey (Ed., & Trans.) *The standard edition of the complete psychological works of Sigmund Freud* (Vol. X). Retrieved from PEP Archives.

Freud, S. (1924). The economic problem of masochism. In J. Strachey (Ed., & Trans.) *The standard edition of the complete psychological works of Sigmund Freud* (Vol. XIX). Retrieved from PEP Archives.

Freud, S. (1938). An outline of psycho-analysis. In J. Strachey (Ed., & Trans.) *The standard edition of the complete psychological works of Sigmund Freud* (Vol. XXIII). Retrieved from PEP Archives.

Frost, R. O., & Shows, D. L. (1993). The nature and measurement of compulsive indecisiveness. *Behaviour Research and Therapy, 31*(7), 683–692.

Gergely, G., & Watson, J. S. (1996). The social biofeedback theory of parental affect-mirroring: The development of emotional self-awareness and self-control in infancy. *International Journal of Psycho-Analysis, 77*, 1181–1212.

Germeijs, V., & Verschueren, K. (2011). Indecisiveness and Big Five personality factors: Relationship and specificity. *Personality and Individual Differences, 50*(7), 1023–1028.

Ginsborg, H. (2014). Kant's aesthetics and teleology. In E. N. Zalta (Ed.), *The Stanford encyclopedia of philosophy* (Fall 2014 Edition). Retrieved from https://plato.stanford.edu/archives/fall2014/entries/kant-aesthetics/.

Glock, H.-J. (1986). Vygotsky and Mead on the self, meaning and internalisation. *Studies in Soviet Thought, 31*(2), 131–148.

Gross, E., Stelzer, N., & Jacob, G. (2012). Treating OCD with the schema mode model. In M. van Vreeswijk, J. Broersen, & M. Nadort (Eds.), *The Wiley-Blackwell handbook of schema therapy* (pp. 173–184). John Wiley & Sons, Ltd.

Hanna, R. (2017). Kant's theory of judgment. In E. N. Zalta (Ed.), *The Stanford encyclopedia of philosophy* (Winter 2017 Edition). Retrieved from https://plato.stanford.edu/archives/win2017/entries/kant-judgment/.

Hansmeier, J., Exner, C., Rief, W., & Glombiewski, J. A. (2016). A test of the metacognitive model of obsessive-compulsive disorder. *Journal of Obsessive-Compulsive and Related Disorders, 10*, 42–48.

Hartmann, H. (1939). *Ego psychology and the problem of adaptation*. International Universities Press, 1958.

Hartmann, H., & Lowenstein, R. M. (1962). Notes on the Superego. In H. Hartmann, E. Kris, & R. Lowenstein (Eds.), (1964). *Psychological issues*. International Universities Press.

Hezel, D. M., & McNally, R. J. (2016). A theoretical review of cognitive biases and deficits in obsessive–compulsive disorder. *Biological Psychology, 121*, 221–232.

Huppert, J. D., Siev, J., & Kushner, E. S. (2007). When religion and obsessive–compulsive disorder collide: Treating scrupulosity in ultra-orthodox Jews. *Journal of Clinical Psychology, 63*(10), 925–941.

Janeck, A. S., Calamari, J. E., Riemann, B. C., & Heffelfinger, S. K. (2003). Too much thinking about thinking?: Metacognitive differences in obsessive–compulsive disorder. *Journal of Anxiety Disorders, 17*(2), 181–195.

Koczanowicz, L. (1994). G. H. Mead and L. S. Vygotsky on meaning and the self. *The Journal of Speculative Philosophy, New Series, 8*(4), 262–276.

Lang, H. (2015). *Der gehemmte Rebell. Struktur, Psychodynamik und Therapie von Menschen mit Zwangsstörungen* [The inhibited rebel. Structure, psychodynamics and therapy of subjects with obsessive-compulsive disorders]. Klett-Cotta.

Lazarov, A., Dar, R., Liberman, N., & Oded, Y. (2012). Obsessive-compulsive tendencies and undermined confidence are related to reliance on proxies for internal states in a false feedback paradigm. *Journal of Behavior Therapy and Experimental Psychiatry, 43*(1), 556–564.

Lazarov, A., Dar, R., Oded, Y., & Liberman, N. (2010). Are obsessive–compulsive tendencies related to reliance on external proxies for internal states? Evidence from biofeedback-aided relaxation studies. *Behaviour Research and Therapy, 48*(6), 516–523.

Leichsenring, F., & Steinert, C. (2017). Short-term psychodynamic therapy for obsessive-compulsive disorder: A manual-guided approach to treating the "inhibited rebel." *Bulletin of the Menninger Clinic, 81*(4), 341–389.

Leopold, R., & Backenstrass, M. (2015). Neuropsychological differences between obsessive-compulsive washers and checkers: A systematic review and meta-analysis. *Journal of Anxiety Disorders, 30*, 48–58.

Longuenesse, B. (2003). Kant's theory of judgment, and judgments of taste: On Henry Allison's Kant's theory of taste. *Inquiry, 46*(2), 143–163.

Luborsky, L. (1984). *Principles of psychoanalytic psychotherapy: Manual for supportive-expressive treatment*. Basic Books.

Mead, G. H. (1964). *George Herbert Mead on social psychology*. Edited by A. Strauss. Phoenix Books, The University of Chicago Press.

Millon, T. (2011). *Disorders of personality: Introducing a DSM/ICD spectrum from normal to abnormal* (3rd ed.). John Wiley and Sons.

Muller, J., & Roberts, J. E. (2005). Memory and attention in Obsessive–Compulsive Disorder: A review. *Journal of Anxiety Disorders, 19*(1), 1–28.

Packer, M. (2018). Is Vygotsky relevant? Vygotsky's marxist psychology. *Mind, Culture, and Activity, 15*(1), 8–31.

Pagacz, K. (2016). *Leaving the OCD circus*. Conari Press.

Parsons, T. (1958). Social structure and the development of personality: Freud's contribution to the integration of psychology and sociology. *Psychiatry, 21*(4), 321.

Pittenger, C., & King, R. (2017). Psychodynamic perspectives on OCD. In *Obsessive-compulsive disorder: Phenomenology, pathophysiology, and treatment.* Oxford University Press. Retrieved February 14, 2021, from https://oxfordmedicine-co m.ezproxy.cul.columbia.edu/view/10.1093/med/9780190228163.001.0001/med -9780190228163-chapter-7.

Rachman, S. (2002). A cognitive theory of compulsive checking. *Behaviour Research and Therapy, 40*(6), 625–639.

Rasmussen, S. A., & Eisen, J. L. (1992). The epidemiology and clinical features of obsessive compulsive disorder. *Psychiatric Clinics of North America, 15*(4), 743–758.

Rassin, E. (2007). A psychological theory of indecisiveness. *Netherlands Journal of Psychology; Dordrecht, 63*(1), 1–11.

Reed, G. F. (1968). Some formal qualities of obsessional thinking. *Psychiatria Clinica, 1*(6), 382–392.

Reed, G. F. (1976). Indecisiveness in obsessional-compulsive disorder. *British Journal of Social and Clinical Psychology, 15*(4), 443–445.

Reed, G. F. (1977). Obsessional cognition: Performance on two numerical tasks. *The British Journal of Psychiatry, 130*(2), 184–185.

Reisberg, D. (2007). *Cognition.* W.W. Norton and Company.

Rieber, R. W. (1997). *The collected works of L.S. Vygotsky: The history of the development of higher mental functions.* Springer US.

Rieber, R. W., & Robinson, D. K. (2004). *The essential Vygotsky.* Springer US.

Salkovskis, P. M. (1985). Obsessional-compulsive problems: A cognitive-behavioural analysis. *Behaviour Research and Therapy, 23*(5), 571–583.

Schafer, R. (1990). *Aspects of internalization.* International Universities Press. (Original work published in 1968).

Schwartz, J. M. (1996). *Brain lock.* Harper-Collins.

Shapiro, D. (2000). *Dynamics of character.* Basic Books.

Stein, D. J. (2002). Obsessive-compulsive disorder. *The Lancet, 360*(9330), 397–405.

Szechtman, H., & Woody, E. (2004). Obsessive-compulsive disorder as a disturbance of security motivation. *Psychological Review, 111*(1), 111–127.

Taillefer, S. E., Liu, J. J. W., Ornstein, T. J., & Vickers, K. (2016). Indecisiveness as a predictor of quality of life in individuals with obsessive and compulsive traits. *Journal of Obsessive-Compulsive and Related Disorders, 10*, 91–98.

Taylor, S., Coles, M., Abramowitz, J., Wu, K. D., Olatunji, B. O., Timpano, K., McKay, D., Kim, S., Carmin, C., & Tolin, D. (2010). How are dysfunctional beliefs related to obsessive-compulsive symptoms? *Journal of Cognitive Psychotherapy, 24*, 165–176.

Tolin, D. F., Abramowitz, J. S., Brigidi, B. D., Amir, N., Street, G. P., & Foa, E. B. (2001). Memory and memory confidence in obsessive–compulsive disorder. *Behaviour Research and Therapy, 39*(8), 913–927.

Tolin, D. F., Abramowitz, J. S., Brigidi, B. D., & Foa, E. B. (2003). Intolerance of uncertainty in obsessive-compulsive disorder. *Anxiety Disorders, 10*, 233–242.

van den Hout, M., & Kindt, M. (2003). Phenomenological validity of an OCD-memory model and the remember/know distinction. *Behaviour Research and Therapy, 41*(3), 369–378.

Voderholzer, U., Schwartz, C., Freyer, T., Zurowski, B., Thiel, N., Herbst, N., Wahl, K., Kordon, A., Hohagen, F., & Kuelz, A. K. (2013). Cognitive functioning in medication-free obsessive-compulsive patients treated with cognitive-behavioural therapy. *Journal of Obsessive-Compulsive and Related Disorders, 2*(3), 241–248.

Wagner, A. P. (2003). Cognitive-behavioral therapy for children and adolescents with obsessive-compulsive disorder. *Brief Treatment and Crisis Intervention, 3*(3), 291–306.

Werner, H. (1948). *Comparative psychology of mental development.* Follett, 1968.

Wilson, A., & Weinstein, L. (1992). An investigation into some implications of a Vygotskian perspective on the origins of mind: Psychoanalysis and Vygotskian psychology, part I. *Journal of the American Psychoanalytic Association, 40*(2), 349–379.

Winnicott, D. W. (1971). The location of cultural experience. In *Playing and reality* (Chapter 7, pp. 95–104). Tavistock Publications.

Winnicott, D. W. (1965). The maturational processes and the facilitating environment: Studies in the theory of emotional development. *The International Psycho-Analytical Library, 64*, 1–276.

Winnicott, D. W. (1960). The theory of the infant-parent relationship. *International Journal of Psychoanalysis, 41*, 585–595.

Winnicott, D. W. (1953). Transitional objects and transitional phenomena: A study of the first not-me possession. *International Journal of Psychoanalysis, 23*(9), 89–97.

Yeomans, F. E., Clarkin, J. F., & Kernberg, O. F. (2015). *Transference-focused psychotherapy for borderline personality disorder: A clinical guide.* American Psychiatric Publishing, Inc.

Index

Aardema, F., 10
Abramovitch, A., 7
aesthetic judgment: political contrasted
    with, 23; in relation to reflective, 21;
    sensus communis in, 28; teleological
    contrasted with, 26
aggression, 112
Allison, H. E., 36n16
ambivalence, 17
apperception, 17
Arendt, Hannah, 23
autonomy: and freedom, 35n13; of
    judgment, 29

Basile, B., 117, 118
beauty, 35n9, 35n12
behavior: compulsive, 56
Beiner, Ronald, 1, 23–26; on reflective
    judgment, 30–32, 102; on *sensus
    communis*, 27; on subsumption, 29,
    35n15
Berk, L. E., 94n5

CBT model of OCD, 4, 5
certainty: Dar on, 10–11, 37; as judgment,
    13–14; OCD limiting, 8–9, 13
checking compulsions, 2–3, 14n1;
    doubt in, 4; memory and, 7; parental
    authority in, 55; uncertainty in, 7

children: ego development in, 96, 98,
    110n10; mothers impacting, 97, 101,
    108; parental authority taken by,
    103; transitional objects of, 98
cleaning compulsions, 3, 14n1;
    hand-washing in, 105; motivation
    of, 105
cognitive self-consciousness (CSC), 8
collective consciousness, 84–85
collective monologue, 83
common sense. *See sensus communis*
compulsions, 2; doubt addressed by,
    3; fear impacting, 3; Freud on, 9;
    as hostile, 15; IU impacting, 5; as
    repetitive, 3; rituals as, 6; ROCD in
    relation to, 33; as self-alien, 116
conclusions, inability to reach, 9–10
confidence: in judgment, 103; in
    memory, 8
consciousness: internalization and,
    81–93; motivation in, 89, 93
"Critique of Judgment" (Kant), 18
CSC. *See* cognitive self-consciousness

Dar, R.: on certainty, 10–11, 37; on
    memory, 8
daydreams: Freud on, 46; and
    introjection, 46; and reality testing,
    47; Schafer on, 46–48

About the Authors

Moshe Marcus graduated from the PhD program in clinical psychology at the CUNY Graduate Center. His theoretical interest has been the exploration of the relationship between psychopathology, clinical practice, and the phenomenology of the self. He is currently completing postdoctoral fellowships at the New York Psychoanalytic Society and Institute and the William Alanson White Institute.

Steven Tuber is professor of Psychology, director of Clinical Training and program head of the doctoral program in clinical psychology at City College, CUNY, where he has taught for over thirty years. He is a diplomate of the American Board of Professional Psychology in clinical psychology, the editor of the book series, *Psychodynamic Assessment and Psychotherapy for the 21st Century* (Lexington Books) and on the editorial board of four different journals, including *Psychoanalytic Psychology and Contemporary Psychoanalysis*. He has authored and/or edited seven other critically acclaimed books and written over 150 papers in the intertwining fields of assessment and treatment of children and adolescents.

www.ingramcontent.com/pod-product-compliance
Lightning Source LLC
Chambersburg PA
CBHW022324280326
41932CB00010B/1220